Care Planning

PEARSON

At Pearson, we take learning personally. Our courses and resources are available as books, online and via multi-lingual packages, helping people learn whatever, wherever and however they choose.

We work with leading authors to develop the strongest learning experiences, bringing cutting-edge thinking and best learning practice to a global market. We craft our print and digital resources to do more to help learners not only understand their content, but to see it in action and apply what they learn, whether studying or at work.

Pearson is the world's leading learning company. Our portfolio includes Penguin, Dorling Kindersley, the Financial Times and our educational business, Pearson International. We are also a leading provider of electronic learning programmes and of test development, processing and scoring services to educational institutions, corporations and professional bodies around the world.

Every day our work helps learning flourish, and wherever learning flourishes, so do people.

To learn more please visit us at: www.pearson.com/uk

David Barrett
Benita Wilson
Andrea Woollands

Care Planning

A Guide for Nurses

Second Edition

PEARSON

Harlow, England • London • New York • Boston • San Francisco • Toronto • Sydney
Auckland • Singapore • Hong Kong • Tokyo • Seoul • Taipei • New Delhi
Cape Town • São Paulo • Mexico City • Madrid • Amsterdam • Munich • Paris • Milan

Pearson Education Limited
Edinburgh Gate
Harlow
Essex CM20 2JE
England

and Associated Companies throughout the world

Visit us on the World Wide Web at:
www.pearsoned.com/uk

First published 2009
Second edition published 2012

ISBN: 978-0-273-74611-9

British Library Cataloguing-in-Publication Data
A catalogue record for this book is available from the British Library

Library of Congress Cataloging-in-Publication Data
Barrett, David, 1972–
   Care planning : a guide for nurses / David Barrett, Benita Wilson, Andrea
Woollands. -- 2nd ed.
       p. ; cm.
   Includes bibliographical references and index.
   ISBN 978-0-273-74611-9 (pbk.)
   I. Wilson, Benita. II. Woollands, Andrea. III. Title.
   [DNLM: 1. Patient Care Planning. 2. Models, Nursing. 3. Nursing Care.   WY
100.1]
   610.73--dc23

                                                        2011050666

10 9 8 7 6 5 4 3 2
16 15 14 13 12

Typeset in 9pt Interstate light by 30
Printed and bound by Henry Ling Ltd, at the Dorset Press, Dorchester, Dorset

To Brid, for everything.
David Barrett

To Drew, with love.
Benita Wilson

With love and gratitude to my family, thank you for your love and support.
Andrea Woollands

Contents

Preface

Welcome to the Second Edition of *Care Planning: A Guide for Nurses*. Being able to plan care for patients is one of the most important parts of your role as a nurse. This book will provide a step-by-step guide to how you can assess your patients, diagnose their problems, plan goals and interventions and evaluate progress. To try to help you use the book, it is worth spending a couple of minutes reading this introduction to the style and layout.

The book is split into two distinct sections. Part 1 deals with the theory of care planning in some detail. The chapters in Part 1 give you an insight into the legal and professional issues related to care planning, the theory of nursing models and the different tools that are in practice to help you assess patients. We will also introduce you to a problem-solving approach to care, based on the nursing process, that we call ASPIRE.

Part 2 is where we put things into practice, with the chapters revolving around ASPIRE. Each part of ASPIRE relates to one step in the process of planning and providing care to your patients, and each chapter will give you information on how it can be done effectively. To help with Part 2, we have provided you with three patient scenarios, which will be referred to throughout the chapters. At the end of the book there are completed care plans for the three patients, which you can refer to throughout the book.

Each chapter has a number of activities for you to complete as a way of building your care-planning skills. Some of these simply involve reading practice examples or research summaries and thinking about how they might relate to your practice. At regular intervals within chapters, we will ask you to stop and think, reflecting on your own clinical practice and the documentation that you use.

There are a number of different terms used to describe the people that you look after in your clinical practice. For example, you may refer to them as patients, clients or service users. We hope you will understand that repeatedly addressing those who require care as a 'patient/client/service user' would be impractical. To try to keep things as simple as possible, we're just going to use 'patients' all the way through the book.

This book has two main aims: first, we hope that it will make clear *why* care planning is so important. Whenever we teach student nurses about care planning, the first hurdle is to try to convince them of the relevance of this to their everyday practice. We hope that, by the time you've read the book, the benefits of assessing patients, planning their care effectively and evaluating progress will be clear.

The second aim is that, by the end of the book, you will have practised the skills involved in care planning. The ASPIRE framework that we discuss in Part 2 should be of real use to you throughout your career as a way of structuring your approach to care.

Just before we finish, it is worth considering possible criticisms of this book. Many people who read it will feel that it is idealistic. There may be comments such as 'We don't have the time to write care plans like this' or 'You never see anything like this in practice.' In some ways, these are fair comments: the book does try to demonstrate 'gold standard', individualised care planning. We recognise that many of you will use core care plans or care pathways, and these are discussed within the book. However, by demonstrating the importance of care planning and showing how it can be done well, you will learn skills that can be used to produce care plans that are fit for purpose – that is, plans that meet your patients' needs and the professional and legal requirements of nursing.

This book is the result of many years of trying to make care planning appear relevant and interesting for student nurses. We hope that we have written a book that you will find informative and accessible, but that is also useful to your own practice.

David Barrett
Benita Wilson
Andrea Woollands

Acknowledgements

We are grateful to the following for permission to reproduce copyright material:

Figure 5.1 from *The Neuman Systems Model, 4th Edition*, Prentice Hall (Neuman, B. and Fawcett, J. 2002). Copyright B. Neuman and J. Fawcett 1970, 1988, 2002. Reproduced with kind permission of the authors.

In some instances we have been unable to trace the owners of copyright material, and we would appreciate any information that would enable us to do so.

Part 1
Care planning theory

Chapter 1
Care planning in context

Why this chapter matters

Imagine that you have just started work on a new ward. You have been given a verbal report for all 32 patients and your head is full of medical terms and abbreviations that no one has had the time to explain to you. All of the regular ward staff are busy elsewhere and you have no idea what you are supposed to be doing. Do you …

1. Continue to flounder for the rest of the shift, not quite knowing what you are doing?
2. Refer to a scrappy piece of paper from your pocket, full of hastily written notes that you made during the report, in an attempt to work out what care each patient requires?
3. Receive a complete picture of each patient that describes their needs, the goals of care, clear instructions on the care to be given and an account of the patient's progress?

It is likely that you have chosen option 3, a choice that gives you the information and guidance that you will need in order to safely and effectively care for your patients. Such a detailed and complex plan may seem an impossible ideal, but with guidance from this book it can be achieved for every patient in every setting. Just think how much easier life would be for student nurses, healthcare assistants and agency staff going to unfamiliar clinical areas if they had all of that information at their fingertips. In addition, registered nurses would know that the members of staff that they were responsible for had a clear understanding of what they were supposed to be doing for each patient.

This chapter will explore why it is so important to develop the skills to plan care and will identify the benefits of care planning for you and your patients. We will demonstrate why care planning should be considered a vital part of your clinical practice and not just an optional extra.

By the end of this chapter you will be able to:

+ outline the difference between care planning and care plans;
+ list two ethical, two professional and two legal reasons why you need effective care planning;
+ identify two things that could improve your own record keeping;
+ give two examples of when the care planning process can go wrong.

Care planning and care plans

One of the problems when discussing this subject is that the terms 'care planning' and 'care plans' are often used interchangeably. They are inter changeable and it is important to clearly identify what we mean by each of these terms. Care planning is the term that is used to describe activities that nurses engage in, from the time a patient is admitted into their care through to when they are discharged. This can be in any setting – acute in-patient, community care or specialist units – and can be for as brief a time as half an hour in an Accident and Emergency department to years for a patient in a care home. The stages of care planning will be explored in detail throughout this book; you may know them as assessing, planning, implementing, and evaluating, sometimes referred to as APIE (Yura and Walsh 1967). In this book we have added two further stages, systematic nursing diagnosis and recheck, giving us an approach that we refer to as ASPIRE (see Chapter 2 for a detailed overview).

Care plans are the written records of this care planning process. There are several methods for recording care, for example **individualised** care plans, core (or standardised) care plans and care pathways; these will be discussed in Chapter 7. Whichever method is used, the care plan is only as good as the person who has written it. Care plans have been criticised by many authors for a variety of reasons, including being difficult to read or understand, being difficult to use, and for not providing enough information about the actual patient care (Allen, 1998; Ferguson *et al*. 1987; O'Connell *et al*. 2000). These criticisms result in nurses and nurse managers questioning the need for care plans. We believe that care plans themselves are not the problem; the issue lies in the way that they are written and used on occasions. Throughout this book we will be suggesting ways to improve the process of care planning and the development of a care plan. Effective care planning is not an optional extra: it is a professional, legal and ethical requirement of your practice. It is for this reason that you need to develop the ability to perform this essential clinical skill. This book provides you with a step-by-step guide.

All nurses should be able to explain their practice; this includes providing an account of what they have done, an explanation as to why they have done it, and an evaluation of the results of their actions. The performance of these actions needs to be documented as an appropriate written record. This is because as a registered nurse you are accountable for your practice; that is, you are held to be personally responsible for the outcome of your own professional actions. There are different levels of accountability: you are ethically (morally) accountable to your patients to do them no harm and to do your best for them; registered nurses are professionally accountable to the **Nursing and Midwifery Council** (NMC), which expects certain levels of professional competence from you; and you are legally accountable not to break the law whilst practising nursing. As a student nurse, you have the same moral and legal accountability as a registered nurse, but your professional accountability differs in that you do not directly answer to the NMC; however you are accountable to your university. The NMC offers guidance on professional conduct specifically for nursing and midwifery students (NMC 2010a).

Individualised is tailored to a specific patient's needs.

Nursing and Midwifery Council is the professional body that regulates nurses and midwives in the United Kingdom.

This book will help you to make your care planning safer and more effective. This chapter will explore the care-planning process and its relationship to your professional accountability and demonstrate some of the pitfalls to be aware of when planning and recording care.

WHAT HAVE YOU LEARNT SO FAR?

+ There are differences between care planning and care plans.
+ Care planning encompasses all that nurses do for a patient, from being admitted into their care to when they are discharged.
+ Care plans are the written records relating to care planning.
+ Care planning and writing accurate care plans are not optional extras but an essential part of nursing.
+ Nurses are ethically (morally), professionally and legally accountable for their actions.

Care planning and professional standards

Care planning and documenting care are essential parts of nursing. They should be considered clinical skills just like administering injections or giving a bed bath, and as such you must be **proficient** in them. Before qualifying, student nurses must demonstrate that they are competent in certain areas of care, as set out by the NMC. The standards for competence (NMC 2010b) cover a wide range of nursing roles and responsibilities, including the ability to carry out key elements of the care-planning process. It's worth looking in more detail at some of these standards to understand just how important care-planning skills are in order to achieve registration as a nurse. Firstly, under the domain of 'nursing practice and decision-making', student nurses need to demonstrate the ability to '...carry out comprehensive, systematic nursing assessments...' and '...plan, deliver and evaluate safe, competent, person-centred care...' (NMC 2010b). In addition to these broad competency statements, the NMC also describes Essential Skills Clusters (ESCs), which outline the different abilities student nurses should have at different stage of their education (culminating with the skills necessary to join the register). The ESCs include many references to care-planning skills, indicating how important care planning is for nurses. Under the ESC of 'Organisational aspects of care', the NMC states that to join the register, a student must demonstrate that she or he: 'In partnership with the person, their carers and their families, makes a holistic, person centred and systematic assessment of physical, emotional, psychological, social, cultural and spiritual needs, including risk, and together, develops a comprehensive personalised plan of nursing care' (ESC 9.12) and: 'Acts autonomously and takes responsibility for collaborative assessment and planning of care delivery with the person, their cares and their family' (ESC 9.13) (NMC 2010c).

Proficient is being able to carry something out competently to a required standard.

The emphasis that the NMC has put on care planning – both in the competency standards and ESCs – demonstrates how fundamental these skills are for delivering high-quality nursing care.

Of course, it's not just about developing these skills as a student – they also have to be maintained and improved throughout your career. *The Code: Standards of Conduct, Performance and Ethics for Nurses and Midwives* (NMC 2008) (we will refer to this as The Code), outlines the standard of professional and ethical conduct expected of you through-out your career; it states: 'You must keep clear and accurate records of the discussions you have, the assessments you make, the treatment and medicines you give and how effective these have been.'

So, for all nurses, care planning is identified as a core skill that you must be able to dem-onstrate throughout your nursing career, from student days until you retire. Student nurses must demonstrate that they have achieved the NMC competencies and skills related to care planning to enable them to register as a nurse. Once registered, if you fail to competently carry out any part of the care-planning process, then you could be removed from the reg-ister. This may sound a bit dramatic, but if you read Practice example 1.1 you will see that it does happen. Current cases of a similar nature can be found at the NMC website, following the links for the conduct and competence committee meetings (www.nmc-uk.org/Hearings/Hearings-and-outcomes/).

Practice example 1.1

A registered general nurse was charged by the Conduct and Competence Committee because of allegations surrounding a failure to assess patients, prepare care plans or eval-uate aspects of care. The nurse had been working as an acting manager of a nursing home.

It was found that a number of patients did not appear to have their needs assessed when they were admitted to the nursing home. One patient, who suffered from diabetes, had a care plan that did not mention the needs related to her pressure ulcers, her diabetes, her mouth care or her pain management. Other patients had care plans that did not address their nursing needs, such as wound care or pain relief.

The committee judged that the nurse should answer for the deficiencies in care, because she was identified responsible and accountable for care planning and patient care. The deci-sion was made to remove the nurse from the NMC register as she had been persistently neglectful over a period of time and had failed to provide adequate records.

NMC (2003)

Accountability and care planning

We have highlighted that there are different levels of accountability, but essentially, it is about being open and transparent about your practice by being able to explain why you have done certain things in a particular way. You are ethically, or morally, accountable to patients to do them no harm (non-maleficence) and to do your best for them (beneficence).

This links to the idea that you have a trust-based relationship with your patients and are therefore bound by ethical principles and values, such as honesty, beneficence, non-maleficence and trust (Beauchamp and Childress 2001). You are professionally accountable to the NMC, which expects certain levels of professional competence and for you to accept the rules and regulations of the profession set out in the NMC Code (Eby 2000). Finally, you are legally accountable – you must not break the law whilst practising nursing and in your personal life, as you may be answerable for your actions through the legal system (NMC 2008).

The Code (NMC 2008) talks specifically about care planning, but it also includes some statements about accountability in nursing and how it links to your responsibilities towards your patients: 'as a professional, you are personally accountable for actions and omissions in your practice and must always be able to justify your decisions'.

This means that registered nurses are answerable for anything that they do (actions) or do not do (omissions) for patients and as such they must be able to explain (justify) their decisions. Good care planning and care plans can help nurses to do this, by demonstrating that decisions about the care were based on comprehensive assessment of the patient, systematic nursing diagnosis, planning of care, evidence-based implementation of care, rechecking and evaluating using a recognised approach. If the care-planning process is followed, the care delivered to patients should be improved, an idea which we will be exploring in this book. The nurse in Practice example 1.1 was removed from the register partly because she did not carry out key elements of care planning: there was no assessment of patient needs, plans for nursing care were not developed and patient progress was not evaluated. Equally, because care plans had not been written, there was no way of knowing whether the appropriate care had been given or not. We will return to some of these issues later on in the chapter when we look at record keeping. The key message at the moment is that, to help you account for the quality of care that you deliver, your care planning and documentation need to be effective.

It is also important to note that registered nurses are accountable not only for their own actions but also for the actions of those that they delegate work to. Therefore, if a registered nurse gives a task to a healthcare assistant or student, then the nurse is accountable for the actions of that person. As care planning is such a complex and important clinical skill and because you are accountable for your actions, only registered nurses should carry out the process without direct supervision. Of course, students need to develop and practise this skill, but should be supervised when care planning, with all documentation countersigned by a registered nurse. This means that if (as a student) you are asked to carry out care planning without direct supervision, you should refuse to do it, because you do not yet have the skills, knowledge or experience to carry out the process effectively or safely. Think of when you are learning to drive: you may be able to control the car and understand the Highway Code, but the instructor has to sit with you all of the time that you are driving until you have passed your test and are then legally considered to be an effective and safe driver. The driving instructor does not say 'I know you can drive; drop me off at the supermarket and you can spend the hour practising on your own'; he has to be in the car with you. Even though you have all the skills to drive, you are not allowed to drive the car on your own until you have passed your test. It is exactly the same as when you are care planning: unless you are a first-level registered nurse, you cannot do it alone. Even if you do have the required skills, you should be supervised during all stages of the care-planning process, including the documentation, to ensure that it is effective and safe. Imagine how you would feel if a mistake was made during the care planning process that affected one of your relatives, and you later discovered that the care had been prescribed following an assessment conducted by a student nurse without supervision. Care planning involves mastering a variety of skills and because of this only registered nurses should be doing it.

WHAT HAVE YOU LEARNT SO FAR?

+ Care planning is a clinical skill.
+ Before qualifying, student nurses must demonstrate that they have achieved specified standards of proficiency set out by the NMC in relation to care planning.
+ You must maintain the standards of proficiency in relation to care plans throughout your career.
+ There are different levels of accountability – ethical, professional and legal.

STOP AND THINK

Think about some of the written records of care that you have seen. Does the documentation give enough information to justify the actions, omissions and decisions?

Making the care-planning process transparent

Unfortunately for student nurses the steps included in care planning and decision making are not always made clear to them. On occasions, registered nurses may carry out the different stages of care planning and make decisions in their heads, often jumping two or three steps ahead of the student who is trying to learn how to do it. Students and unregistered staff need to have all of the steps of the process clearly defined so that they can learn how decisions have been made. The purpose of this book is to make all of the steps involved in care planning transparent to you; this should make the process easier to learn. However, it is not only students who would benefit from care planning becoming a more transparent process; it would also benefit all patients, staff and the organisations that employ them. Also, patients are more likely to understand, give their consent to and comply with their plan of care if they understand how it has been developed.

If a registered nurse fails to write a clear care plan or adequately document relevant information, it is difficult for members of the team to work without clear directions of what they are expected to do for patients. For registered nurses, this may pose less of a problem, as they can draw upon their experience and knowledge to decide on how best to care for patients. However, if the practitioner's care were to be questioned at a later date, it would be difficult to justify their decisions and actions without adequate written records.

One of the major issues to consider when care planning is the actual framework used to guide the process. The approach chosen must provide a systematic framework that can be used by all of the nurses in a given clinical area, to provide a consistent, comprehensive and accurate account of care planning for each patient. The approach used most often in the UK is a combination of the problem-solving process (APIE) and a nursing model. Throughout this book we will explore an adaptation of the problem-solving process, which we call ASPIRE (see Chapter 2), in conjunction with the Activities of Living Model by Roper, Logan and Tierney (2000), the Self-Care Model of Nursing by Orem (2001), and the Systems Model by Neuman (2010b). Students are sometimes told by clinical staff that the care planning used in an area is based on a named model, but then the model is not used correctly or not applied to all the stages of ASPIRE. This is confusing for students, other staff and patients when using the care plan. To maintain consistency, it is essential for all nurses to follow the approach accurately to ensure that aspects of care are not overlooked.

There are several reasons why the care-planning process should be transparent. Patients are not cared for by the same nurse all of the time, so all of the nurses caring for a patient need access to the same information as the nurse who assessed the patient and wrote their care plan. If care is challenged (for example, a complaint is made about the care), a transparent process will provide the details of the care and also the evidence for how decisions about the care were reached; this protects both the nurse and the organisation that they work for. Students and other unregistered staff need to have all the steps of the process clearly defined, so that they can learn how decisions have been made.

WHAT HAVE YOU LEARNT SO FAR?

+ The care-planning process should be transparent for the patient, staff and others.
+ Care planning should be underpinned by a framework to guide the process.

Care planning as a way of improving patient care

As stated earlier in the chapter, one of the reasons for using this book is to develop your care-planning skills in order to improve the care provided for your patients. One of the reasons why you need to develop these clinical skills is that it is vital that the care-planning process leads to safe and effective care. A failure to recognise patient needs or to deal with their identified needs can lead to detrimental consequences for the patient. It is therefore essential that the whole care-planning process is comprehensive. We will be exploring these ideas throughout the book, but Activity 1.1 demonstrates some of the issues with failing to recognise or deal with patients' needs.

Activity 1.1

Mrs Curtis, a 67-year-old woman, is admitted to a medical ward with a suspected **deep vein thrombosis (DVT)**. Having been weighed, Mrs Curtis realises that she has lost 6 kg (nearly a stone) over the past three months; she was not overweight before, and is now under her ideal weight. The nurse conducting the assessment goes to the office to complete a care plan, and selects a pre-printed core care plan for patients with weight loss. On this pre-printed plan are instructions to refer the patient to a dietician, and this is duly done by the nurse. Mrs Curtis is surprised a few days later to be visited by the dietician to discuss her dietary intake.

Talking to the nurse after the dietician's visit, Mrs Curtis says that she had a nice chat with the dietician, but that she didn't really need to see her as she knew about the information that she had been given, having been a domestic science teacher before she retired. On closer questioning about the weight loss, it is found that Mrs Curtis' husband died three months ago and that due to this her lifestyle has completely changed. From being an active, fit and highly sociable woman, eating a healthy diet, she has become a virtual recluse, seeing very few people, giving up her exercise and not eating well as she 'couldn't be bothered to shop for food or cook for one'.

There has been a lack of communication between the nurses and Mrs Curtis, resulting in needs being overlooked. What could have been done to improve the care that Mrs Curtis received and make it more patient-centred?

How did you do? The example in Activity 1.1 raises a lot of important points about care planning. First, we need to think about the assessment that took place; it seems that the nurse found out about Mrs Curtis' weight loss but did not look for the cause. There are many reasons why patients may lose weight: there could be physical reasons such as illness or difficulty in preparing and/or eating food; there could be psychological reasons such as eating disorders; there could be social or environmental reasons such as low income or lack of access to shops. The nurse had not found out that the weight loss was due to lifestyle changes following her bereavement, and this affected the way in which the nurse dealt with the problem. The nurse failed to establish that the weight loss was not due to a lack of knowledge about nutrition, because she failed to find out what Mrs Curtis' occupation was before retirement. In the first step of the care-planning process – assessment – the nurse had not asked Mrs Curtis about many aspects of her life; the assessment lacked detail about the psychological and social factors that might have been the cause of the problems. This means that the assessment was not comprehensive and therefore the whole process was made less patient-centred and was more likely to lead to an incorrect plan of care for the patient.

Even if a comprehensive assessment has been completed, it is important to document all of the relevant information about the patient, so that the details of their lifestyle are available to the rest of the healthcare team. We look at assessment in more depth in Chapters 2 and 8, suggesting ways that you can make your care planning comprehensive and therefore safe and effective.

Deep vein thrombosis (DVT) is a blood clot in the leg.

Activity 1.2

Are the assessments that you have observed in practice comprehensive? Could you identify patients' needs and the cause of those needs from the documentation?

Activity 1.2 raises a number of ethical and professional issues. Ethically, Mrs Curtis in Activity 1.1 did not receive the best possible care and failure to identify the cause of her needs (an omission in care) could have put her at further risk. You have a responsibility to yourself and the patient to give the best possible care that is professionally competent, effective and legally safe. Professionally, in Activity 1.2 the nurse did not fulfil the obligation to give the best possible care, did not set a good example for student nurses and wasted the time of a fellow professional, the dietician.

In the case of Mrs Curtis, no real harm was caused as a consequence of the nurse's failure to identify the cause of her weight loss. Unfortunately, however, there are occasions where omissions or actions in the caring process can lead to harm. Harm that occurs as a direct result of something the nurse did do (action) or did not do (omission), and that could be reasonably foreseen, may lead to a nurse being sued for negligence. (For further details of negligence, see Dimond 2011.) To try to illustrate this, Practice example 1.2 shows where a failure in the care-planning process has a much more serious effect on the well-being of a patient.

Practice example 1.2

A student nurse reported to her mentor that she had noticed the heels of an 87-year-old woman were red and dry. The ward used core care plans, but the student could not find one for prevention and treatment of pressure sores. The mentor, a first-level registered nurse, said not to worry about the lack of a core care plan; when the student said she would write an individualised plan for the need, she was told that it was too time-consuming. The student was concerned about this, as it was her last day on the ward, but she did not want to upset her mentor. Although she did not feel able to write a needs statement, goals and interventions required to reach the goals, she did record the state of the patient's heels in the nursing notes, which the mentor then countersigned. The following day the mentor, a staff nurse, went on annual leave for two weeks.

Returning to the ward two weeks later the staff nurse found that the patient had developed a **gangrenous** heel and had surgical **debridement** to remove the dead tissue. The patient was now in a lot of pain and the whole incident resulted in her discharge being substantially delayed.

Gangrenous is the tissue which has died due to lack of blood supply.

Debridement is a procedure to remove damaged tissues, dead cells, foreign bodies and dirt from wounds.

Activity 1.3

Now that you have read Practice example 1.2, think about the following questions:

1. Is there a case for negligence here?
2. Who was responsible for the patient developing pressure sores and why?

How did you get on with Activity 1.3? In this case it could be argued that the patient suffered from **foreseeable harm** as a direct result of omissions in care, and the nurse could therefore be deemed negligent. A number of things went wrong here. The registered nurse was informed by the student nurse that the patient was at risk but failed to act appropriately (in other words, this was an omission in her care). Although the student recorded that the patient's heels were red, a plan of care identifying the problem, setting goals and planning suitable interventions was not written for the potential problem of developing pressure sores. There was a failure to comply with her duty as a nurse to keep proper and accurate records (NMC 2009a). Even though the patient was already at risk, there is a big difference between red heels and serious pressure sores. Other nurses on the ward failed to observe the patient adequately and note the pressure sore until it had developed considerably, meaning that the information in the nursing notes was not used, and a full and accurate plan of care for the potential problem of pressure sores was not developed.

The responsibility for the development of pressure sores lay with the registered nurses on the ward, the mentor who dismissed the student's concerns and those who failed to observe the patient's pressure areas effectively. As a direct result of these omissions in care, the patient suffered from foreseeable harm. Even if no negligence case was brought against the nurse, the nurse could still be answerable to the Conduct and Competence Committee of the NMC. If the decision of the committee is that the nurse is guilty of misconduct and her fitness to practise is impaired, a number of sanctions can be made, including being permanently removed from the register (Dimond 2011).

Practice example 1.2 demonstrates that it is not just about giving the appropriate care, but about documenting the care process accurately and comprehensively in order to demonstrate to everyone that the care has been delivered. If the student and her mentor had written a plan of care to deal with the risk of pressure sores (or even used a core care plan), and if this plan had been followed, then the sores may not have developed. We believe that improved care planning leads to improved care, and that this book can help enhance your skills in this area.

Foreseeable harm is harm that could have been reasonably predicted as occurring if an action did or did not occur.

WHAT HAVE YOU LEARNT SO FAR?

+ As a nurse, you are professionally and legally accountable for your actions and omissions.
+ When producing a care plan, you need to ensure that it is comprehensive and individualised.
+ If a problem is identified, then it is essential that a plan is developed to deal with this problem appropriately and all actions are documented.

Care-planning documentation

Earlier in the chapter we identified why the care-planning process has to be transparent. The first reason was that patients are not cared for by one nurse but by many nurses, and everyone caring for that patient needs to share the relevant information. The only way to do this is to document the information; it cannot be shared with others if it is in a nurse's head or if it is part of a brief conversation between two nurses. If you think about your own personal life, you tend to write down important information so that you do not forget; you do not rely on your memory in order to remember dentist appointments and birthdays: you write them down on a calendar. This means that family members can share the information too. In your professional life, everything about patient care is relevant, so all the details about the care should be written down to ensure that there is no breakdown in communication and that important things are not forgotten. Care plans should provide a working document that allows the nursing team to care for a patient safely and effectively without the need for lengthy and time-consuming verbal handovers. By documenting care effectively you can help to improve outcomes through recording important information about patients' health and their responses to nursing care (Jefferies *et al.* 2010).

Chapters 2 and 8 will explore why we need to conduct an accurate and comprehensive assessment of patients. Many nurses are very good at obtaining information from patients; unfortunately not all nurses then document it so that it can be shared by the nursing team. This information is crucial to the rest of the care-planning process in order to diagnose, plan, implement, recheck and evaluate the care that the patient receives. Not only do the patient and the rest of the team need this information but also, if the care is challenged, it needs to be made clear to the organisation that you work for, to your professional body (the NMC) and possibly to a court of law how decisions about care were made. As seen earlier with Mrs Curtis, the assessment was heavily biased towards information about the physical factors affecting her, and psychological and sociological information was not obtained. This is something that has been noted time and again by the investigations into complaints by the **Health Service Ombudsman**. In these investigations it has been found that the emphasis is on

The **Health Service Ombudsman,** also known as the Health Service Commissioner (HSC), investigates complaints about the National Health Service (NHS) in England. The service provided by the HSC office is free and is independent of the NHS. It acts impartially and can effect positive change within the health service. (See Dimond 2011 for further information.) (www.ombudsman.org.uk)

information of a medical nature and about the physical aspects of the patient. Information about the patient's view of their care and about psychological, social and spiritual aspects is often missing. This means that the assessment is not comprehensive or patient-centred. In Chapter 8 it will become clear why this has such important consequences for the rest of the care-planning process.

The NMC document *Record Keeping: Guidance for Nurses and Midwives* (NMC 2009a) makes it clear that you 'should record details of any assessments and reviews undertaken, and provide clear evidence of the arrangements you have made for future and ongoing care. This should also include details of information given about care and treatment'. The National Health Service Executive (NHSE) (1999) also suggests that 'the purpose of health records is to ensure those coming after you can see what has been done, or not done and why and by whom'.

NMC guidelines give clear instructions on the way you should write your records. This deals with issues such as making sure that you do not use jargon, ensuring that entries are dated and signed, and making sure that they are legible. NMC guidelines make clear that good record keeping can, amongst other things, promote high standards and continuity of care and allow for improved communication between healthcare team members. They also highlight how important it is to write accurate records so that your care can be assessed by other people months or years after you delivered it. If your nursing documentation is ever looked at in a professional hearing or a court of law, then the approach taken will be that if it is not recorded, it has not been done'. The NMC (2009a) also states: 'Good record keeping is an integral part of nursing and midwifery practice, and is essential to the provision of safe and effective care. It is not an optional extra to be fitted in if circumstances allow.'

Once the assessment has been done (see Chapters 2 and 8), a nursing diagnosis, followed by the planning of care, needs to be documented (see Chapters 9 and 10); this should be done with the patient. If the patient is involved with every step of care planning, then they are far more likely to follow the plan of care in order to reach their goals; this is called compliance (or concordance) with treatment. Patient involvement will help the care to be much more focused on the patient's wishes and choices. Patient choice has been embedded in successive UK government White Papers (Department of Health [DH] 2004, 2006), culminating in the principle of 'no decision about me, without me' in the most recent White Paper, 'Liberating the NHS' (DH 2010). Also, planning care with the patient means that it is far more likely that you will have the patient's informed consent for the care that they will receive – an essential step, ethically, professionally and legally. The activities that are required to reach the goals should be written in a way that leaves no room for misunderstanding (see Chapters 2 and 10). All nurses, the patient and other healthcare professionals should understand their contribution to the care of the patient. It is no good simply writing that you should follow 'procedure 112', as the patient and other nurses may not know what that means. Each instruction for care has to be written out in full, making it clear and comprehensive. A test of good documentation is to ask yourself the following question:

If I was an agency nurse who didn't know this clinical area or this patient, would I understand exactly what care I had to provide to the patient today by reading the care plan?

Writing out instructions for care in full may seem time-consuming and, when certain activities are repeatedly carried out in a clinical area (for example, preoperative care on a surgical ward), it is perfectly acceptable to use a core care plan, as long as it is personalised for each patient (see Chapter 7). In the Ombudsman's reports of investigations into complaints made by patients, there are constant referrals to the lack of a plan of care being recorded, which means that there was no information for the staff about the management of the patients' problems (see the examples at the end of this chapter).

Once care has been given to patients, it is essential to record the results. Evaluation is a crucial part of care planning (see Chapter 12) as it enables the patient and the nurse to establish how effective the interventions have been – that is, whether the goals of care been achieved or not. Without evaluation and the accurate recording of outcomes, it would be difficult to ascertain whether or not nurses and nursing were making a difference. This is very important at the present time, as the numbers of nurses are reduced and non-nurses are doing what were once considered to be nurses' jobs. If – as nurses – we cannot demonstrate that what we are doing is essential for the patient, then we are in danger of making ourselves unnecessary.

From an ethical perspective, care needs to be recorded to enable the patient to see what has been planned and what progress has been made. From a professional perspective, all nurses caring for the patient need access to all of the information about the patient and an accurate record needs to be kept to ensure that professional standards are upheld (NMC 2008). From a professional and legal perspective, if records are used in complaints and negligence cases, there is a view that poor record keeping may reflect poor care. This is why it is essential to accurately record the whole of the care-planning process from assessment to evaluation as soon as possible after it has happened. If you fail to do this, you may be at risk of losing your nursing registration. We have seen in the case of Mrs Curtis (Practice example 1.1) how an incomplete assessment can lead to inappropriate care being given. Practice example 1.2 shows the importance of why patient information needs to be communicated effectively and how patients can suffer if this is not done. It is because of the serious problems that can be caused by poor care planning and documentation that the NMC insists that it is done well.

RESEARCH SUMMARY 1.1

Diana Jefferies and colleagues carried out a meta-study of quality nursing documentation. A meta-study is essentially a piece of research that gathers together and analyses the findings of previous studies on a particular subject. This allows you to identify themes that come from the whole evidence base, rather than just an individual piece of work.

They looked at 28 articles related to nursing documentation and identified 7 'essentials' of quality record keeping:

1. Nursing documentation should be patient-centred.
2. Nursing documentation must contain the actual work of nurses including education and psychological support.
3. Nursing documentation is written to reflect the objective clinical judgement of the nurse.
4. Nursing documentation must be presented in a logical and sequential manner.
5. Nursing documentation must be written contemporaneously, or as events occur.
6. Nursing documentation should record variances in care within and beyond the health-care record.
7. Nursing documentation should fulfill legal requirements.

Jefferies D, Johnson M, Griffiths R (2010) A meta-study of the essentials of quality documentation. *International Journal of Nursing Practice*. 16: 112-124.

The rest of this book will expand on the themes identified in this chapter and help you to improve your documentation and care planning skills.

When the care-planning process goes wrong

It should now be evident why the care-planning process needs to be comprehensive, transparent and accurately documented for the benefit and understanding of patients and staff. However, it may also be necessary for people outside your workplace to understand the process. In particular, if the standard of the care that you provide is ever challenged, for example by a patient or their family, then your records will be scrutinised to ensure that care is properly documented and that the reasons for your decisions are clear. During the period 2008–2009 almost one in twelve of all allegations reported to the Conduct and Competence Committee of the NMC related to failure to maintain adequate records and the consequences for those cases proven varied from removal from the register to supervised practice (NMC 2009b). Let's consider a case of a nurse who appeared before an NMC Conduct and Competence Committee in 2011. The case was based on a number of failings in care, but most of the charges centred on record keeping – here's just one of the charges:

> *This charge relates to inaccurate record keeping. High standards of record keeping were required under the registrant's job description and also under the NMC code of professional conduct, keeping clear and accurate records. The registrant failed to accurately record entries in Patient C's evaluation of nursing care record, community nursing communication sheet and a fax to Patient C's GP. Such inconsistent entries could have had an impact on the planning and delivery of patient care. The panel therefore regards her actions as serious failings which amount to misconduct.*

This demonstrates how seriously the NMC treats breaches in record-keeping guidance and professional practice. In this nurse's case, the decision of the panel was to give a caution order for five years.

Another organisation that may review your nursing documentation if a complaint is made is the Health Service Ombudsman. Within Ombudsman investigations, there are regular references to the poor standard of care planning and documentation.

Sometimes, it is reported by the Ombudsman that nursing assessments are biased towards information related to physical factors and medical problems; we have already identified this oversight in the case of Mrs Curtis (Practice example 1.1) and how this can cause problems in the rest of the care-planning process. Other times, the Ombudsman reports that the documentation itself is not as good as it should be, and it sums up the importance of good documentation in a statement that outlines how nurses 'should include the items of information and education provided to patients in the clinical record – not for defensive purposes, but to assure effective communication between health care professionals' (Health Service Ombudsman 2000).

In one specific case the Ombudsman looked at the care of a patient with **myeloma**. In this case, the patient (Mr J) was diagnosed with advanced myeloma and underwent chemotherapy to try to treat the disease. Despite this, his condition quickly worsened, he developed kidney failure and he died soon after. The Ombudsman investigation raised a number of issues about the clinical care that was given to Mr J, and it made a number of recommendations. In the course of the clinical investigation, the nursing notes were looked at and criticised. The Ombudsman found that 'the nursing documentation on the first ward was scant and there was no evidence to suggest appropriate nursing care planning or careful monitoring of Mr J's condition' (Health Service Ombudsman 2005).

In other words there was no way of knowing whether Mr J had been cared for properly because nobody had documented the assessment, systematic nursing diagnosis, planning, implementation, recheck and evaluation of care. The Ombudsman report went further: Mr J was, in the course of his final hospital stay, transferred from the first ward (a general medical ward) to a specialist haematology ward, where, once again, nursing documentation was poor. It was found that:

There were no written care plans and no written protocols documented either on the patients' notes or in separate reference folders which staff could then access. Therefore, there was nothing to provide information or supportive prompts for any of the staff, whether trained, untrained, regular, or bank staff, to assist them in caring for haematology patients.
(Health Service Ombudsman 2005)

STOP AND THINK

Next time you are at work, look at care plans and nursing progress notes for your patients. Ask yourself the following questions:

+ If I was an agency nurse who didn't know this clinical area or this patient, would I understand exactly what care I had to provide to the patient today?
+ If I looked at my nursing documentation months after the care episode, would I be able to explain and justify what care was planned and given?

If the answer to either of these questions is 'no', then the records need improvement and enhancement to ensure that they are fit for purpose. This book will help with that process.

Myeloma is a malignant disease of the bone marrow.

The Ombudsman report about Mr J is by no means unique in highlighting poor nursing documentation and the problems that this can cause. You have a professional obligation to maintain patient records to a high standard; failure to do so could result in poor patient care and even disciplinary proceedings.

Conclusion

This chapter should have helped you to understand why care planning and care plans are so important; in other words, it should have given you some idea why this book will be useful to you in your nursing career. As a registered nurse, it is essential that you are proficient at care planning. If you are a student, you should take any opportunity that you have to prac-tise the skill, so that you are ready to do it on your own once you have qualified.

In order to carry out care planning effectively, it is essential that the whole process is comprehensive, transparent and accurately recorded. As a nurse you are responsible and accountable for your own practice and for the safety of your patients. This will improve patient care, enhance communication between healthcare practitioners and ensure that any complaints about care can be investigated more thoroughly.

Care planning is an essential skill for all nurses; this book will help you to learn and practise the skill. To help make the process as clear as possible, we will introduce a problem-solving approach to care planning in the next chapter and then explore the process in more detail in the second part of the book, using patient scenarios. Try to have a go at the tasks that we have set so that you can practise your care-planning skills in a safe environment. The best way to learn to ride a bike is by getting on and practising, carrying on even when you fall off. Telling you how a bike works, how to pedal or recalling our experiences may help, but the real learning and development of the skill comes from you having a go and refining your attempts. In this book, we are just providing the stabilisers, so go and have fun.

Further reading

NMC *Record Keeping: Guidance for Nurses and Midwives (2009a)*. You can find this on the NMC website at www.nmc-uk.org

NMC Code: *Standards of Conduct, Performance and Ethics for Nurses and Midwives (2008)*. This can also be found on the NMC website at www.nmc-uk.org/aFrameDisplay.aspx? DocumentID=3954

If you want to read more about accountability and issues surrounding the importance of record keeping, try *Legal Aspects of Nursing* by Bridgit Dimond (2011).

Finally, if you are a student of nursing and midwifery, then you need to ensure that you have read and understood the NMC guidelines set out for your professional conduct, which can be found at – http://www.nmc-uk.org/Documents/Guidance/NMC-Guidance-on-professional-conduct-for-nursing-and-midwifery-students.pdf

Chapter 2
ASPIRE – the problem-solving approach to care delivery

Why this chapter matters

If you had to cook for your family tonight, where would you start? If we assume that taking everyone for a curry or getting a pizza delivered is not an option, you will need to devise a plan to guide you. By being organised and planning ahead, you will be able to cook a nutritious, cost-effective, enjoyable meal for your guests.

First, you will have to think about the needs of the family, their likes and dislikes based on previous experiences and present preferences, whether they want to eat together or whether they are all demanding different meals at different times. You will also need to consider the resources that are available to you to help you deal with the task, such as how much money you have to spend, what foods are in season and whether you have the time to shop at the supermarket or high street. In other words a thorough *assessment* of the circumstances and situation would have to take place. Once this stage has been completed you will need to devise an action plan; this could involve choosing a recipe and identifying a list of ingredients, which will then guide the *planning* of a shopping list. A trip to the supermarket to buy the food and the final act of cooking and serving the meal would complete the *implementation* of your plan. However, it is not over yet; you may want to spend some time establishing how effective your approach has been in meeting the individualised needs of the family members. Perhaps you could ask questions about whether they have enjoyed the meal, or whether they feel full and satisfied. Part of this *evaluation* will probably involve you considering and making a mental note of the effectiveness of the approach in meeting the family's needs; you might look at the plates to see if anything was left and maybe ask them if they have any suggestions for improvements. All of this information will be stored and used the next time you have to make a meal for the family, with the cycle of assessing, planning, implementing and evaluating starting all over again.

This process offers a useful approach to anyone who finds themselves confronted with a problem that requires a solution. The example that we've looked at relates to your personal life, but the problem-solving approach is also crucial in your professional life when you are trying to help a patient deal with a health need. This chapter will therefore explore the problem-solving approach to care, and show how it relates to your everyday work.

By the end of this chapter you will be able to:

+ explain the theory and philosophy underpinning the problem-solving approach to care delivery;

+ list the six stages of ASPIRE;

+ list the key elements of the six stages of ASPIRE.

The nursing process

The process of assess, plan, implement and evaluate (which is abbreviated to APIE in the clinical area) was introduced to nursing by Yura and Walsh in 1967. It was called 'The Nursing Process', and it attempted to direct nursing practice away from intuition and ritual practice, in a hope that nurses would start to use a more structured systematic approach. In other words, rather than just doing things because 'they've always been done that way' or because 'it seems a sensible thing to do', nurses would start providing care that was based on the best evidence and on the individual needs of their patients.

The term 'nursing process' has come in for some criticism, because it suggests that only nurses carry out the process of APIE, but this is certainly not the case. As illustrated at the start of the chapter, the process can be used as a logically sequenced set of steps to deal with any problem and forms the basis of decision making in the working practice of many other professions. It is for this reason that we shall refer to the 'problem-solving approach to care'. The four stages of the approach form the basis of the NMC competency standards for students that we explored in Chapter 1 (NMC 2010b). Consequently, demonstration of an ability to assess, plan, implement and evaluate in the clinical setting is what underpins many of the practice learning outcomes in current nurse education programmes. Whether you are a student or registered nurse, it is therefore vital that you are clear about what happens at each of the stages.

It is true to say that the original format of APIE has been modified and refined over the years and this chapter offers a user-friendly exploration of the stages to help direct your practice in the clinical setting. The descriptions are based on the ideas of APIE as described by Yura and Walsh (1988), but we have expanded the explanations and suggested extra stages within the process, which we have named ASPIRE. These changes and additions should help you understand the steps a little better and recognise how they can help you in practice.

ASPIRE

One of the weaknesses of the original nursing process is that only four stages are identified; this means that two elements of the problem-solving approach are missing. The first of these is systematic nursing diagnosis, which occurs between the assessment and planning stages. It is a systematic process by which patients' problems are identified and a nursing diagnosis is made. The second missing element is what we call recheck. This is the process by which the nurse gathers and then documents the information that you need in order to evaluate whether the implementation of care is proving successful. It is about monitoring the patient's situation or condition as it changes (or not) following the implementation of the pre-scribed care. We also encourage the use of baselines which personalise and clarify the patient situation, and offer an explanation of what experienced practitioners do during the stage of evaluation to make the task more transparent and understandable for novice nurses.

We are not suggesting that the nursing process is wrong; we simply feel that important elements of a problem-solving approach have not been identified as clearly as they could be. To remedy this, we suggest that when using the problem-solving approach you make use of the stages of ASPIRE rather than APIE. ASPIRE consists of six stages in a cyclical pattern, as shown in Figure 2.1.

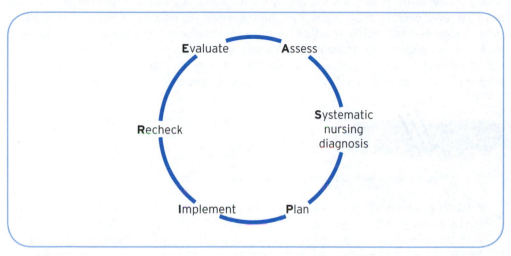

Figure 2.1 ASPIRE

Assessment

Assessment or admission?

At some point in your working day, particularly if you work in a hospital or nursing home, you will be asked to 'admit' a patient. It is important to say at this stage that assessment is not the same thing as admission. The terms are often used in the clinical setting to mean the same thing, but although they are related, they are in fact very different activities.

Admission is about introducing yourself to the patient and, if not nursing them in their own home, making them feel comfortable and welcome in their new environment. This includes dealing with any immediate needs they may have that you can deal with. This might involve helping them get changed, making sure they have a jug of water available, and show-ing them where they can find the call bell and toilets. You can start the assessment process by gathering very basic information such as name, age, date of birth, next of kin and even vital signs, but this is by no means all that assessment should involve.

Assessment is a much more complex process than admission and therefore should only be undertaken by a registered nurse or by a student supervised by a registered nurse. The other thing that separates assessment from admission is *when* it is carried out. Admission tends to be a one-off process when you first meet the patient, whereas assessment carries on throughout your relationship with the patient.

What is assessment?

Assessment is not about listing problems; it is as much about finding out what the patient can do as it is about finding out what they cannot do. Assessment is a multi-stage procedure that produces a detailed representation of the patient. It should offer a true likeness of them as an individual, highlighting their needs (present and near future) and the resources they have available to deal with these needs. Insight into their usual routines and ways of dealing with their everyday life and problems should be included in the description.

A good detective never makes a decision as to who has committed the crime until they have gathered every possible detail from the scene and the individuals involved. If Sherlock Holmes identified the murderer without a thorough assessment, the risk of a criminal walking free or an arrest of an innocent person would be a real possibility. If a nurse fails to carry out a systematic, comprehensive assessment or relies on the patient's diagnosis to list the problems, they may well identify the wrong problem or overlook a concern altogether.

STOP AND THINK

Read through the scenario for Suzy Clarke (see Appendix A).

What do you think about Suzy and her panic attacks? If the nurse had made a list of Suzy's problems rather than conducting a detailed assessment, the fact that she is drinking large amounts of cola (which contains caffeine) might have been missed. One of the ways of dealing with Suzy's panic attacks would be to help her develop strategies to cope with the experience, but the nurse would also need to advise Suzy about reducing her caffeine intake – because it can mimic the signs and symptoms of panic or make them worse. If a systematic, comprehensive assessment is not conducted, then the nurse may well identify the wrong problem or overlook a concern altogether, making the original situation much worse.

What should an assessment find out?

During an assessment, it is not appropriate to write 'no problems' in the description. Instead, a comprehensive assessment that offers an objective, accurate, detailed account of the individual and their life must be conducted. Think about a good Agatha Christie novel; all the information for identifying the crime and solving the murder is in the text of the book. In a thorough assessment, all the information for identifying the needs, planning, implementing and evaluating the care should be present in the description. Miss Marple's ability to make sense of the information and solve the crime at the end of the book is very much dependent upon her using her assessment and analysis skills. In much the same way, the nurse has to engage in similar skills to conduct a systematic, comprehensive assessment of a patient and these will be discussed later. Consider Activity 2.1.

Activity 2.1

Read the scenario for Suzy Clarke. It is clear that Suzy has thrush (*Candida albicans*) as diagnosed by her general practitioner. What would you need to find out about the thrush to help her deal with the problem more effectively?

If you are carrying out a holistic assessment of Suzy's needs, you shouldn't just write down the diagnosis and medical treatment. In order to assess Suzy's needs comprehensively, you will have to consider the following:

+ What is she normally like?
+ What is she like now?
+ Is there a change or difference?
+ What has caused the change or difference?
+ What is she doing about it?
+ What is anyone else doing about it?
+ What resources does Suzy have (or had in the past) to deal with the problem?

Remember: when you gather the information you will need to be as accurate and clear as you possibly can be. You are trying to establish the actual problems (things that are causing the patient difficulty now) and any potential problems (things that might cause the patient problems in the future because of their illness or because of any treatment that they might undergo). Activity 2.2 will help you recognise the difference between actual and potential problems.

Activity 2.2

James is a 55-year-old male admitted to hospital for a hip replacement. He is receiving a patient-controlled **analgesic (morphine)** to help reduce his postoperative pain. He is not allowed out of bed for the first 24 hours, but he will gradually increase his mobility until he is partial-weight bearing on his operated hip, using crutches. If everything goes to plan he will be discharged in five days' time. Can you identify James' actual and potential problems in relation to his pain?

Analgesic is a drug that relieves pain.

Morphine is a strong analgesic, belonging to the opioid family.

How did you do with Activity 2.2? The actual problem is that James is experiencing pain. However, he is also at risk of a number of potential problems such as constipation, nausea and vomiting due to the morphine, inflammation or swelling at the site of the **intravenous cannula**, and pressure ulcers due to his reluctance to move because of the pain and enforced bed rest. As a nurse, it is not enough to identify problems that already exist; it is also important that you anticipate problems that might occur in the near future.

WHAT HAVE YOU LEARNT SO FAR?

+ During an assessment, you should find out what is 'normal' for a patient, in terms of their routines, habits and behaviour.
+ The assessment process allows you to build up a picture of the patient's health problems, how they are coping with them (or not), and what the possible causes might be.
+ Previous and present resources that are available to deal with the problems need to be identified.
+ A good assessment should be able to identify actual problems and any potential problems.

What are the skills that are needed for assessment?

Assessing a patient effectively requires you to use a number of different skills. These include:

+ interviewing or talking to the patient or relatives and friends to obtain information;
+ observing or looking for signs that offer information about the patient such as their general appearance and home environment, whether their skin is flushed or discoloured, and non-verbal communication:
+ measuring things such as height, weight, blood pressure and levels of pain;
+ inferring or using evidence to reach a conclusion – for example, if a patient is rubbing their back and wincing every time they move, you would probably infer that they were in pain;
+ identifying or recognising information that describes the patient's circumstances or condition;
+ discriminating or 'filtering' information to try and decide what is significant and what is less important;
+ analysing or taking very complex information, breaking it down into its individual parts, examining the issues and then reaching a considered conclusion.

An **intravenous cannula** is a small tube inserted into a vein, through which fluids and medication can be administered.

What are the possible sources of information?

The focus of assessment is to collect information (sometimes called data). You are expected to gather this information from a variety of sources, so it is important to identify exactly what you are looking for.

Subjective data, sometimes known as qualitative data, is descriptive information that relates to the quality of the patient experience. This is the sort of information that you will get if you ask somebody 'How do you feel?' or 'What is worrying you?' Sometimes, your own skills may add subjective data to the overall assessment; for example, you may think that a patient seems 'very withdrawn and uncommunicative'.

Objective data, sometimes known as quantitative data, is information that can be measured, such as vital signs, blood results and weight, but could include scores from fear and worry scales.

Together these can offer a rich account of the patient's circumstances that will prove invaluable when you come to the later steps of planning care.

Subjective and objective information can be obtained from a number of different sources, such as the following:

+ Repeated information: information offered directly by the patient and family members as well as other healthcare workers. This might include biographical information (e.g. name, date of birth, address and next of kin) and insight into things like normal routines and present concerns.

+ Observed information: information that can be gathered by observing the patient. This might include information such as the colour of mucous membranes in the mouth, the condition of a patient's skin, or their ability to walk and move. Observing the patient may also give you some useful information about the way they interact and communicate with others.

+ Clinical information: this might include vital signs, medical diagnosis, blood results, X-ray or scan results, and the results of assessment and treatment by other healthcare workers such as physiotherapists and occupational therapists.

Have a go at Activity 2.3.

Activity 2.3

Look again at the Suzy Clarke scenario in Appendix A. Can you identify some examples of objective and subjective information about Suzy? Compare your answer with the assessment included in the care plan.

Please be careful: it is important that you are aware when assessing a patient that many factors can influence the experience and outcome for both you and the patient. These are some of the factors:

+ ability to make use of sensory information – vision, hearing, smell, touch;

+ physical state – tiredness, illness, stress, hunger, hormone levels;

+ psychological state – knowledge base, cognitive abilities, emotion, motivation, perception of information and events;

+ social and cultural background;

+ use of language – verbal and non-verbal.

STOP AND THINK

Read the text below:

OPPORTUNITYISNOWHERE

What did you see? 'Opportunity is now here' or 'Opportunity is nowhere'? It is clear that the same information can be perceived differently; explanation for the difference may be due to one or more of the factors already discussed. Do any of them help explain why you perceived it the way you did?

The process works in two ways: the factors that can influence the nurse can also influence the answers that you receive from the patient and their family and friends.

Making sense of the information

Once all the information is collected, it needs to be collated in a manner that the healthcare team can understand. It can be presented in the clinical area in many formats, depending on the nursing model and form of documentation used by the team. The formats for assessment and collation that can be used to create a care plan will be discussed in more detail in Chapter 7.

Whatever type of documentation is used, the information that you write down will provide the starting point for you and your colleagues to identify actual and potential needs, and ensure that the rest of care planning goes smoothly.

Of course, though there is an ideal method of assessment, putting this into practice can sometimes be challenging. The research example below highlights some of the barriers to comprehensive and holistic assessment, and describes how these barriers cause problems in practice.

RESEARCH SUMMARY 2.1

Jones (2007) observed or taped 72 nursing assessment interviews on a total of five hospital wards. When the contents of these interviews were analysed, they demonstrated that assessment was not always the idealistic, patient-centred, valued part of the care-planning process. Instead, assessment interviews were often seen as an onerous part of the nursing role, structured according to the documentation used and focused on completing paperwork, rather than providing the basis for planning nursing care.

The study raised real concerns about nursing interviews with patients, and highlighted the need for greater understanding of the importance of a comprehensive, holistic and patient-centred approach to assessment.

Jones A (2007) Admitting hospital patients: a qualitative study of an everyday nursing task. *Nursing Inquiry.* 14(3): 212-223

> ### WHAT HAVE YOU LEARNT SO FAR?
>
> + The main activity of assessment is to collect information or data.
> + There are two types of information – subjective/qualitative and objective/quantitative.
> + The information gained during assessment can take many different forms, such as repeated information, observed information and clinical information.
> + It is important that you take care during the assessment process, and recognise that many factors can influence the experience and outcome for both the patient and nurse.
> + Once all the information is collected, it needs to be collated. Once all the assessment information is documented, it should allow you and your colleagues to identify actual and potential problems, providing a starting point for the other stages of care planning.

Systematic nursing diagnosis

Practitioners and theorists writing about the problem-solving approach do not always identify nursing diagnosis as a separate task, instead 'bundling in' diagnosis with assessment. However, this can make it difficult for nurses to understand the complexity of developing an accurate nursing diagnosis. Equally, using only the four-stage APIE approach to care planning means that the nurse does not have time to reflect on the assessment process before moving on to the planning stage (Hogston and Marjoram 2006). Adding the stage of systematic nursing diagnosis offers you direction and quality time to reflect on what the patient's problems are and – through a systematic approach – develop a nursing diagnosis. This is necessary because nursing problems are often overlooked; this is not surprising when you consider how many theorists have struggled to offer a definition of nursing diagnosis, not least because it is often confused with medical diagnosis.

Systematic nursing diagnosis involves identifying the patient's needs from a nursing perspective. It is important to recognise that nursing diagnosis and medical diagnosis are not the same thing. Nursing diagnosis differs from a medical diagnosis because it places the emphasis on the holistic needs of the patient by considering the physical, psychological, social and spiritual consequences of 'owning' a collection of signs and symptoms or a particular medical diagnosis. The problems that you identify may be linked to the medical diagnosis, but others will arise from the psychological, social and spiritual issues related to living with the illness or disease. Nursing takes into account the consequences of living with the signs and symptoms but also how the patient interacts with others, such as family and friends and their environment (Christenson and Kenney 1995). It then follows that nursing intervention is more than treating signs and symptoms: because it is not just the illness or disease that requires nursing care, we need to adopt a holistic approach.

Consider Activity 2.4.

Activity 2.4

Can you offer a nursing diagnosis for the following patient?

Zaheer Kahn is a 54-year-old male who had a **myocardial infarction** three days ago. He is very anxious and frightened about the future and is worried about all the drips, monitors and leads that he is attached to.

How did you do with Activity 2.4? There is no doubt that a large part of the nurse's role is to monitor Zaheer's heart rhythms, ensure that he receives the prescribed medication and make sure that he receives the care prescribed by other healthcare professionals. However, the systematic nursing diagnosis would also consider the individual, holistic needs that arise from having a myocardial infarction. In other words, the systematic nursing diagnosis would address the fact that Zaheer is anxious and frightened about the future and is worried about the technical care that he is receiving.

Once you have carried out a systematic nursing diagnosis, you need to write a clear statement identifying the patient's nursing needs. This statement is called different things depending on what nursing model is being used, but we will refer to them as need statements. They should be written in a way that the patient and their carers can understand; this means that there should be no medical jargon or abbreviations. For example, if you work in a GP practice and a patient comes to see you because of the headaches that are keeping them awake, then a need statement for this patient could be 'Mr Jones is having trouble sleeping due to headaches'.

Simple, isn't it? However, did you notice the difference between this need statement and the type of medical diagnosis that you might see in the patient notes? A medical diagnosis would focus on the medical problem 'suffering from headaches'. The nursing diagnosis should focus on how the medical problem is affecting the patient's life: in this case, by stopping Mr Jones from sleeping.

Alongside the need statement there should be some baseline information. A baseline offers a description or measurement of where the patient is now in relation to the need, and helps you to personalise the problem. The baseline is used when evaluating the patient's movement towards or away from the goal; therefore, it should be a clear description of the situation or circumstance as it is now. A simple example that demonstrates the importance of baselines is weight loss: if you have ever gone on a diet, the first thing that you will do is to find out how much you weigh before you start the diet. If you do not do this, you will have no idea whether or not the diet has worked. The baseline will allow you to see at a glance if you have lost weight or put weight on.

Myocardial infarction is death of heart muscle cells, usually caused by a blood clot in a coronary artery.

You shouldn't have to find out anything new to write your baselines, but you will need to highlight the relevant information from your assessment. So, let's go back to Mr Jones and his headaches. Now that you have identified that his headaches are causing him problems sleeping, we need to look at the assessment that you have done and 'cherry-pick' the baseline information that is relevant. These baselines will include a combination of objective and subjective information. For Mr Jones, the baselines may include how long he sleeps at the moment, the quality of his sleep, a description of the pain and how frequent the headaches are.

By this stage, our care plan will include need statements and relevant baselines. The final thing that we need to do is decide in which order to deal with the different needs; in other words, we need to prioritise. This process should be patient-led, although you may have to seek advice from the patient's relatives or friends if the patient is unable to act or do for him or herself. Sometimes, needs are prioritised because of obvious safety issues: if a patient is bleeding from a wound, you will deal with that before worrying about their constipation. On other occasions, the patient themselves may request that certain issues are handled with greater urgency than others. Have a look at Activity 2.5.

Activity 2.5

Can you write a need statement and a baseline for Suzy Clarke in relation to her panic attacks? Compare your answer to the care plan in Appendix A. Did you include all the key elements?

WHAT HAVE YOU LEARNT SO FAR?

+ Systematic nursing diagnosis involves identifying the patient's needs from a nursing perspective.

+ Systematic nursing diagnosis differs from medical diagnosis because it places the emphasis on the holistic needs of the patient that arise from owning a particular set of signs and symptoms or medical diagnosis.

+ Once a nursing diagnosis has been made, a clear, short statement concerning the patient's needs is identified along with baselines.

+ The patient should have ownership – the need statement should be written using terms that the patient can understand.

+ A baseline offers a description or measurement of where the patient is now in relation to the need; they personalise the problem.

+ The baseline is used when evaluating the patient's movement towards or away from the goal.

+ Finally the needs are prioritised – a process that should be patient-led.

In some clinical areas, the need statement and nursing diagnosis are seen as the same thing, but it is our belief that systematic nursing diagnosis is the process that you have to go through to identify the need statements. We will be exploring how you can carry out this process in the second half of the book, where the difference between systematic nursing diagnosis and need statements will become clear. However, it may prove useful to look at the difference between making a nursing diagnosis by luck or instinct and one that uses your clinical decision-making skills in a systematic way.

To try to demonstrate this, have a go at Activity 2.6. This has got nothing to do with nursing, but it does demonstrate the systematic approach to diagnosis.

Activity 2.6

It's an unseasonably warm December morning and you are about to set off to work in your car. Unfortunately, when you turn the key in the ignition, nothing happens apart from a whining noise. You last used the car the previous evening when you picked it up from having a service and filled it up with petrol.

What do you think the problem might be?

How did you do? The first thing that you should have done is read the scenario to gather evidence; in other words, you should have carried out an assessment. You then needed to move things on to the next stage by attempting to systematically diagnose the problem. In order to do this you would have to analyse the data. This involves a number of different steps: first of all you break down the information into smaller parts; you should have been able to identify a number of possible reasons from the assessment as to why the car did not start.

+ The car is out of petrol.
+ The battery is flat.
+ The engine is not starting because the weather is too cold.
+ The starter motor is not working.

Whilst these are all feasible causes, you need to continue to analyse the data in more depth and move on to the next step, to quickly rule out some of the possibilities. The scenario told us that it was a warm December day, so the temperature is probably not the cause. The car was picked up from the garage after a service yesterday, so the starter motor should be fine. It was also filled up with petrol the day before, which rules out the first possibility. All we're left with then – our most likely problem – is the option that the battery is flat. We can test this idea by looking at the most likely reason for a flat battery: the lights being left on. Indeed, a quick look reveals that the switch for the lights has been left in the 'on' position. Therefore, the reason that the car won't start is that the battery is flat because the headlights were left on overnight. This is what is known as a differential diagnosis because the process allowed you to consider all the possible causes and rule out each one before deciding on the most likely cause.

Finding out why the car would not start involved a systematic approach to allow you to arrive at a diagnosis by a process of reductionism – reducing the many possible causes to one possible answer. This approach is similar to the process used by your doctor when identifying what is wrong with you. To discover the most likely cause of your problem, they consider all the possibilities of what it could be, then engage in a process of differential diagnosis, before arriving at the most likely cause of your signs and symptoms; this reductionist approach then offers a medical diagnosis. The medical diagnosis or label defines your illness, usually from a biological stance.

Systematic nursing diagnosis is different to medical diagnosis because nurses need to go beyond identifying the most likely cause or medical diagnosis. Nurses have to consider the signs and symptoms or medical diagnosis and then establish all the needs that arise as a consequence of living with these. This means that we don't reduce the problem to its smallest possible cause. What we do is expand on the initial diagnosis or signs and symptoms to include all the possible problems associated with the medical label. We also consider how the problems are interrelated and are interdependent. 'Interrelated' refers to establishing which of the problems are related to each other – if the patient had a diagnosis of common cold the related problems could be temperature, sore throat, runny nose and loss of appetite. 'Interdependent' refers to establishing how the problems are dependent on each other – inability to sleep and loss of appetite are related problems because they are dependent on the cold getting better; as the cold improves the problems will subside. This needs to occur because nurses need to look at the patient from a holistic perspective rather than a reductionist approach, thereby nursing the patient and not the medical label. If we go back to the example of the car, systematic nursing diagnosis would equate to working out the problems that will arise as a consequence of the car not starting. It may be that you will be late for work, you won't be able to pick up the children from school; you won't be able to go to the shops for the food for dinner tonight; or you will not be able to afford to pay for a new battery.

We have spent a long time discussing how we got from 'The car won't start' to 'I'm going to be late for work because I left the lights on and the battery is flat'. In reality, this process would probably take place quickly and the same may be true when carrying out a systematic nursing diagnosis for a patient. It is often possible for nurses to develop diagnoses extremely quickly and without apparent effort because of their knowledge and expertise. Even if it is not apparent, a systematic approach is still being used:

+ An assessment is taking place using theoretical knowledge and past expertise.
+ Analysis is taking place and possible problems are being identified.
+ Critical thinking is allowing identification as to how the problems are interrelated and interdependent
+ Critical analysis allows a conclusion to be made by establishing the nursing diagnosis, based on the consequences of living with the signs and symptoms or medical diagnosis.
+ Synthesis allows a need statement and baselines to be written to reflect this nursing diagnosis.
+ The nursing diagnosis is confirmed by going back to the patient to clarify that the problems have been included in the need statement and that it represents their experience.

However, when this process is not transparent or obvious, a novice nurse can struggle to understand how the experienced nurse is arriving at their nursing diagnosis.

Finally, it is worth spending time looking at how nursing diagnosis is addressed in North America. The reason for doing this is that there is a much more formalised approach to nursing diagnosis in North America than in the United Kingdom and it is different from the approach and explanation that we are offering you.

An organisation called the North American Nursing Diagnosis Association (NANDA) is one of many that develops updates and classifies nursing diagnoses that are used in practice in America. These diagnoses are defined, risk factors for each are listed and detailed characteristics are included. This is best demonstrated with an example from the NANDA list, which you can find in Practice example 2.1.

Practice example 2.1

Nursing diagnosis: Body image disturbance.

Related factors: Include physical trauma, pregnancy, maturational changes.

Defining characteristics: Include verbal or non-verbal negative response to actual or perceived change in structure and/or function, preoccupation with change, not looking at body part, hiding body part, self-destructive behaviours.

Adapted from Carpenito (2000)

At first the diagnosis and the supporting information in Practice example 2.1 seem very different to what we are proposing. However, it is similar in that it is not a medical diagnosis and it still attempts to focus on the holistic consequences of living with the body image disturbance.

Planning

This next stage of ASPIRE involves the making of a care plan: the nurse identifies goals and prescribes the care that will meet the patient's needs. The crucial thing to remember is that the patient is central to this process, which means that a partnership between you and the patient needs to be established. Within this partnership, a contractual agreement is made, whereby care delivery is patient-centred and individualised. This approach features in professional recommendations and is essential if the goals are to be realistic and achievable. Imagine having to write an essay as part of an academic programme, but finding that all the guidelines are in a language that you cannot understand and the lecturer does not explain the task or refer to it during your teaching sessions. This is what it must seem like for some patients when goals are written using medical terminology and jargon that they do not understand. Also, if the care plan is kept at the nurses' station or in the ward office, making access impossible, it is not surprising that the patient fails to progress as much as the nurse would like.

Setting goals

The purpose of setting goals is to help you and the patient solve or alleviate problems and, where possible, avoid potential problems from becoming actual problems. Goals should offer a short, directive statement as to the outcome of the nursing care. If a baseline is where the patient is now in relation to the problem, a goal is where they should be as a result of the nursing care. Depending on the patient and their needs, the goals can be short- or long-term; however, it is often better to set short-term goals as a way of maintaining motivation and morale.

At some point the nurse and patient will have to evaluate whether the problem is getting better by moving towards the goal or getting worse by moving away from the goal. Therefore, goals should be simple, achievable, measurable, achievable, and recordable and devised within the limits of the available resources to deal with the problem. It may help you when you are writing the goal to consider the following:

+ Who is meant to achieve the goal?
+ What are they meant to achieve?

+ How are they meant to do it?
+ When are they to do it by?

Criteria for setting goals

There are different criteria available to help nurses write patient-centred goals, one of which is MACROS – Measurable, Achievable, Client-centred, Realistic, Outcome-written and Short (Hogston and Marjoram 2006), but an alternative way to remember what you need to include is to use the word PRODUCT, which directs you to write goals that are:

+ **P**atient-centred – is the goal tailored to the patient's needs?
+ **R**ecordable – can you document the progress towards the goal?
+ **O**bservable and measurable – can you evaluate the progress?
+ **D**irective – is it clear who, what, when and how?
+ **U**nderstandable and clear – is it written in a simple way?
+ **C**redible – can it be realistically achieved by the patient?
+ **T**ime-related – when is the goal meant to be achieved?

Now try Activity 2.7.

Activity 2.7

Write a goal for Suzy in relation to her panic attacks; remember to use the PRODUCT criteria. Compare your attempt with the care plan in Appendix A; did you include all the elements?

WHAT HAVE YOU LEARNT SO FAR?

+ Planning is about making a care plan, identifying a goal and prescribing the care.
+ The patient is central to this two-stage process, which means that a partnership between the nurse and the patient needs to be established.
+ The purpose of setting goals is to solve or alleviate problems and, where possible, avoid potential problems from becoming actual problems.
+ A contractual agreement is made, whereby care delivery is patient-centred.
+ Goals can be short- or long-term.
+ Goals should offer a short, directive statement as to the outcome of the nursing care.
+ Goals should be simple, achievable, measurable, and recordable and devised within the limits of the available resources to deal with the problem (time, nursing staff, equipment etc.).
+ There are criteria that help nurses devise patient-centred goals, such as PRODUCT.

Prescribing the care

Once you have identified and agreed the goals with the patient, you then need to prescribe care based on the most up-to-date research and evidence. The care is in the form of activities that you, your colleagues, the patient and their family carry out to achieve the goals. The prescription offers a set of logically sequenced instructions that direct the actions of the patient and carers. The plan should resemble a recipe, in the sense that it should offer clear, unambiguous directions that, if followed, will lead to the successful completion of the task – that is, the achievement of the goal. As with any recipe, you need to make sure that the instructions are also in order – you cannot put the icing on a cake until you have taken it out of the oven. Therefore, it is important that you start with the first step that needs to be taken and end with the last step, which is usually an instruction to evaluate the care.

The plan for implementing care should direct the patient and their carers as to who is to deliver the care, what they are meant to do, when are they meant to do it, and where they are meant to do it (if appropriate). You should also be able to offer an explanation as to why the care is the most effective choice and provide evidence to support this, although you wouldn't be expected to write this in the care plan. For example, if you are writing a prescription of care for a patient with constipation, can you explain why you have recommended an increase in fluids, fibre and exercise? Is the practice based on evidence or research? Is the plan safe, legal and ethical? These are the types of question that need to be considered when prescribing care.

The prescription may include actions that reflect the directions of other healthcare professionals or address the consequences of the treatments prescribed by them. For example, a doctor may prescribe pain relief, but it is the nurse that needs to ensure that the patient is given the medication and monitored for side effects and tolerance to the drug. The nurse will also have to consider the potential problems that arise from taking the pain control, such as constipation, nausea or diarrhoea.

In the assessment stage, you were asked to find your patient's coping strategies or ways of dealing with their everyday life and problems. This information needs to be used when the prescription of care is devised. Wherever possible, nursing actions need to be organised around current or individual behaviours, as it is often easier to modify an existing behaviour than to substitute a new one. Whatever the actions, they need to be consistent with the goal and be within the scope of the available resources. Consider Activity 2.8.

Activity 2.8

Think about the Suzy Clarke scenario and her diagnosis of thrush (*Candida albicans*). The scenario outlines the care that she needs, but can you write a prescription of care that includes who, what, where and when?

How did you do? Did your prescription of care include Suzy in the directions? Is it clear what all the people involved in her care should be doing? Does it help Suzy cope with the problem?

WHAT HAVE YOU LEARNT SO FAR?

+ The prescription offers a set of logically sequenced instructions that direct the actions of the patient and caregivers.

+ The directions should include details of who, what, when and where (if needed).

+ You should prescribe care that is based on research and evidence.

+ It is important to start with the first step that needs to be taken in the procedure and end with the last step, which is usually an instruction to evaluate the care.

+ You should be able to offer an explanation as to why the care has been prescribed and be prepared to answer public, professional and legal questioning in relation to the care.

+ The prescription may contain actions that meet the directions of other healthcare professionals and also the consequences of the treatments requested by them.

+ The prescribed care needs to be consistent with the goals and be within the scope of the available resources.

Implementation

By this stage, you will have carried out a comprehensive assessment, made a nursing diagnosis, set some individualised goals with the patient and prescribed the care to be given. Implementation is the next stage of ASPIRE; this is the 'doing' part of the care plan, where the prescription of care is put into action and actually carried out. It would be impossible to discuss all the possible actions that the nurse and patient may be involved in during this stage. This is partly because of the sheer volume of actual and potential problems that you will have to deal with, but also because there will be cultural and individual differences that will affect the way in which the care is delivered. An individual's values and beliefs will influence what they are willing to do or allow you to do for them. Some patients would not hesitate if you offered to bathe them, but would be unhappy for you to choose a menu or prepare their drinks and meals. Others would insist on washing themselves at all costs, even if it meant that all they could do was wipe their own face, although they would be content for you to prepare their drinks and food. Equally, there are individuals from certain cultures that need to bathe in running water and would find it uncomfortable if they were made to take a bath. There are many cultural restrictions and considerations in relation to food preparation and presentation that may have to be acknowledged, in order to individualise the delivery of the care you give (Baldwin *et al.* 2003).

STOP AND THINK

Think about your own experiences when you are unwell and in need of care. What actions would you expect the nurse to do for you and what actions would you like to do for yourself? Would you want any of the actions to be carried out in a very specific way?

It is very easy to fall into the routine of implementing the care in a standardised way, which is delivering the same care to all patients without taking individual and cultural differences into account. *The Code: Standards of Conduct, Performance and Ethics for Nurses and Midwives* (NMC 2008, p. 1) requires nurses and midwives to 'make the care of people your first concern, treating them as individuals and respecting their dignity'. This cannot be achieved unless we make sure that we embrace the diverse cultural and individual differences in our patients.

Many nursing models offer a description of the activities that a nurse and patient may be involved in during this stage and some of these will be outlined in Chapter 11. It is true to say that there are certain considerations that need to be at the forefront of your mind when you are implementing care. These are as follows:

+ Is the care individualised and patient-centred?
+ Is the care safe, legal and ethical?
+ Is the care based on evidence or research?
+ Are the resources necessary to deliver care – knowledge, skills, staff and equipment – available?
+ Was consent obtained in order to carry out the plan of care?
+ Was dignity and respect for the patient maintained at all times?
+ Were the actions consistent with the prescribed care – in other words, did you follow the instructions accurately?
+ Did you communicate with the patient, their carers and your colleagues in an effective and considerate way about the care?
+ Were the actions documented in accordance with the relevant organisational and professional guidelines and policies?

You will have noticed that a lot of these considerations relate back to the prescription of care that you produced during the planning phase. This underpins the key message that this book is trying to deliver – a good care plan can help make your actual nursing care more effective and safe.

WHAT HAVE YOU LEARNT SO FAR?

+ Implementation is the 'doing' part of the nursing process.
+ There is a range of different ways of implementing care, and the approach you use will be governed by the clinical area, the nursing diagnosis, and the patient's individual needs and preferences.
+ Many of the models of nursing give a description of the activities that a nurse and patient may be involved in during this stage.
+ There are a number of core principles that you should consider when delivering nursing care.

Recheck and evaluation

Traditional views of evaluation

The final stage of APIE is evaluation (Yura and Walsh 1967). There are two types of evaluation with which you will be involved within the practice setting and many nursing models refer to these as formative and summative (Roper *et al.* 2000; Neuman 2010b) .

Formative evaluation

According to Yura and Walsh (1967), formative evaluation involves you and the patient deciding whether the problem is getting better or worse. It is the patient's behaviours or activities that become the focus for the evaluation of this progress. However, the process must involve the patient and consider their experiences; after all, they are the experts on themselves.

Yura and Walsh (1967) suggest that the purpose of formative evaluation is to see whether the patient has progressed towards or moved away from the set goal. The task involves you considering the information that you have available to you and making a judgement as to whether the patient has achieved each of the goals. This highlights the importance of making sure that the goals are clearly written so that they can be used to evaluate the patient's progress on the date decided by you and the patient. When the goals have not been achieved, the process does not end; what happens is that you need to restart the problem-solving process of APIE and repeat the stages until the need is addressed. In this sense the process is cyclical, suggesting that there is a continuous flow from one stage to the next; the end stage (evaluation) can often lead us back to the beginning stage (assessment). It is also important to note that even if goals have been achieved in the desired time, there are questions that still need to be asked at this stage. The sorts of questions or concerns would be: Has achieving the goal solved or alleviated the problem? Were the goals too easy for the patient? Was there an awareness of potential problems? (Roper *et al.* 2000). Have a look at Activity 2.9 and consider some of these issues in more depth.

Activity 2.9

Think about Suzy Clarke and her problem of thrush. How would you carry out a formative evaluation? List the possible sources of information that could be used in your evaluation.

Summative evaluation

Summative evaluation is when the effectiveness of the process and general approach to care is evaluated. Consideration is given towards whether the assessment was comprehensive and holistic, and whether the assessment led to an accurate nursing diagnosis that was then defined as patient-centred need statements and baselines. Time is devoted to establishing whether the set goals were realistic and relevant and whether the prescribed care was appropriate in terms of meeting the goals. Issues of documentation and record keeping in relation to the patient's progress are considered, so that an accurate, comprehensive evaluation can be made of how effective the approach has been.

Consider Activity 2.10.

Activity 2.10

Think about Suzy Clarke and her panic attacks. How would you conduct a summative evaluation of her experience? List the possible sources of information that could be used in your evaluation.

How did you get on with the formative and summative evaluation for Suzy's goals? Yura and Walsh (1967) offer a simple, uncomplicated, logical stage that addresses the achievement of goals and provides clear information for audit purposes. However, our experience of helping nurses understand the care-planning process is that they do not find this last stage as straightforward as it would first appear. The main comment is that it is too vague and not as directive as they would like it to be; questions such as 'What information would I need to help me evaluate?'; 'How do I detect deterioration or improvement in the patient's condition if I do not evaluate until the formative evaluation date?' are often asked. It is because of questions like these that we have introduced an extra stage named 'recheck', as well as offering clarification of what experienced practitioners do during the different stages of evaluation. We have already explained that we are not saying that the nursing process is wrong; our rationale for suggesting extra stages and further clarification is to make the process transparent and useable, especially for novice nurses.

Recheck

Without rechecking the patient's situation and evaluating their progress, there is no real way of knowing how successful your care has been. Let's think about a simple example from life: changing a light bulb. After assessing the situation and discovering that the light doesn't work, you make a diagnosis (the light is not working), set yourself a goal (to get the light working) and prescribe an intervention (replace the light bulb). Once you have done all this and changed the bulb, what is the first thing you do? You switch the light on to see if it is now working; in other words, you recheck the situation. With the information that you get from rechecking, you can then evaluate whether or not you have achieved the goal. If the light works, then your intervention was a success and the problem is solved. However, if the light still does not work, then your intervention has failed and the problem remains. This will mean that you will have to restart the problem-solving approach.

What is rechecking?

Rechecking is about gathering and documenting the information that you need in order to evaluate whether the implementation of care is proving successful. It is about monitoring the situation as it is now and describing and documenting the patient's progress to date. It can involve the skills of interviewing, observing, measuring and identifying, as discussed in the assessment stage. Rechecking should not be seen as 'reassessment' because rather than the comprehensive assessment process that we discussed earlier, it is the gathering and monitoring of very specific and targeted information linked to a specific problem. For example, let's assume that a patient has pain. You assess the patient's pain, reach a systematic nursing diagnosis, develop a goal related to the relief of the patient's pain and then prescribe and implement care. After a defined period of time, you go back to the patient and find out how their pain is now by asking them the appropriate questions and recording their descriptions and pain ratings; this is rechecking. Even if the recheck stage involves taking a blood pressure, temperature or recording of a blood result, the process is still one of describing and documenting the progress to date using the information that you have available to you. It's important to recognise that recheck does not require any judgements to be made regarding how well the patient is progressing – that happens during evaluation – but simply requires data collection, description and documentation. The nursing process, or APIE does not include 'recheck' as a distinct stage; Yura and Walsh (1967) describe formative evaluation as a stage that includes collecting information to help make the decision as to whether the goal has been achieved or not. The reason that we feel it is worthy of inclusion in the process of ASPIRE is because it is different to evaluation and occurs throughout the episode of care rather than during the last stage of the care-planning cycle.

Have a go at Activity 2.11.

Activity 2.11

Think about some of the patients you have looked after recently. List five activities that you carried out that could be classed as 'rechecking'.

How did you do? We hope that by now you will have started to think about the vast amount of rechecking that you do each day for your patients. The sorts of activity that you have identified could include measuring vital signs (such as blood pressure and pulse), establishing pain scores, talking to the patient about how they feel or measuring fluid intake and output. If there is deterioration from the baseline reading, you would report the change to the nurse in charge because a reassessment of the situation is required. Essentially, anything that you do at work that enables you to monitor and document a patient's condition can be seen as rechecking.

WHAT HAVE YOU LEARNT SO FAR?

+ Rechecking relates to the process of gathering information.
+ It is the gathering of very specific and targeted information linked to a specific problem and goal.
+ It provides an opportunity to highlight deterioration to baseline readings that you would need to report to the nurse in charge.
+ Where there is deterioration to the baseline readings, it is reported to the nurse in charge as a reassessment of the situation is required.
+ The process of rechecking involves you describing and documenting the patient's present condition and progress to date – a crucial element of care that underpins subsequent evaluation.

Ongoing and final evaluation

There are several reasons as to why we have proposed the adaptations and additions to the APIE process – including documenting baselines in the care plan, adding the extra stage of systematic nursing diagnosis and redefining the evaluation stage. Formative evaluation (Yura and Walsh 1967, Roper *et al.* 2000, Neuman 2010b) doesn't really emphasise baselines and their role in evaluation, despite being crucial to this stage. You cannot really make an informed decision as to whether there has been movement away from a goal without the use of a baseline; nor can you really make a judgement in relation to the degree of progress your patient has made. Without a baseline the best you can do is to comment when the patient has actually achieved the goal, but using a baseline allows you to make a judgement as to the degree of progress and effectiveness of the prescribed care. This suggests that without the use of baselines it is difficult to identify deterioration but also early achievement of the goals. That is why we propose that nurses engage in recheck and what we call 'ongoing evaluation'.

Formative and summative evaluation (Yura and Walsh 1967), as adopted by most of the nursing models (Roper *et al.* 2000, Neuman 2010b), don't really help you deal with goals that have a very short time frame. If we were to set a goal and evaluate according to the principles of formative and summative evaluation for a patient recovering from anaesthetic or in relation to the effectiveness of oxygen therapy on their oxygen saturation levels, we may find ourselves reassessing and setting several goals over a very short time, because the patient's condition is changing rapidly. However, ongoing evaluation addresses this issue, making it possible to set one short-term goal that calls for changes in behaviour over a short time, but allowing us to detect deterioration or improvement without having to write several goals.

What is ongoing evaluation?

Ongoing evaluation involves a registered nurse and the patient deciding whether the problem is getting better or worse based upon the patient's behaviours, activities and other findings from the recheck phase. It is an ongoing decisive activity, where a registered nurse makes a decision about two key factors related to their patients. First, by considering baselines in relation to goals and recheck information, ongoing evaluation allows nurses to judge the patient's movement towards or away from their goals – that is, their progress. This then allows the nurse to make judgements regarding the effectiveness of the care itself – the process. A clinical decision is then made as to whether the prescribed care is to be continued or not, and whether any changes need to be made.

When evaluating progress, you may find that the patient is improving, with movement towards (or even early achievement of) a goal. Alternatively, there may be a change from the baseline that demonstrates deterioration. This would require a more detailed assessment to identify whether there was an explanation for this, or why the prescribed care was not having the desired effect. For example, Matt is recovering from a recent knee operation two days ago. On return from theatre his pain was recorded as 6 (this is his baseline) and his agreed goal is that the pain will be reduced to 2 by 28.11.12. During the recheck of his current condition you record his pain levels and document that it has increased to 7, you then notify the nurse in charge because there is deterioration beyond the baseline of 6. The registered nurse carries out an ongoing evaluation in response to the deterioration to the baseline by considering the patient's progress in response to the prescribed care (process). He notes from the care plan that the recheck information was gathered 10 minutes after the physiotherapist finished helping Matt with his exercises and therefore makes the clinical decision to continue with the prescribed care and goal. Pain control is offered and recheck is carried out 30 minutes later to allow the nurse in charge to carryout ongoing evaluation. Equally, if there is a change from the baseline that demonstrates that the goal has been met before the stated time frame, the care could be discontinued, unless the change is only a temporary improvement and the treatment needs to be continued. For example, Gino has been admitted to the recovery ward following a repair of an inguinal hernia. The care plan asks you to check his vital signs every 15 minutes for the first hour, every 30 minutes for one hour, hourly for two hours then four-hourly (this is an example of rechecking – describing and documenting his progress to date). His baseline reading in theatre is 95/65mmHg and his goal is that his blood pressure will be 110/70mmHg by 4 p.m. on 5.11.12. On the third recheck at 12 p.m. you notice that Gino's blood pressure has returned to the pre-operative reading of 110/70mmHg and therefore he has met the goal earlier than anticipated. The registered nurse carries out the ongoing evaluation as usual at the end of the morning by considering Gino's progress in response to the prescribed care (process), but she does not document that the goal has been achieved. This is because she acknowledges that the recheck process was carried out when Gino was laid flat, but he now wants to get out of bed to pass urine and it is time for him to sit up and have a drink. She makes the clinical decision to continue with the prescribed care and goal. Ongoing evaluation will be repeated at 2 p.m. or in response to deteriorations to the baseline as identified in the recheck stage.

Ongoing evaluation involves critical analysis of the information, rather than a description of the situation or condition as seen in the stage of recheck, and must involve the patient and consideration of their experiences.

What is final evaluation?

The purpose of final evaluation is to see whether the patient has achieved the goal on the date identified in the planning stage and whether the experience was right for them as an individual. This cumulative task requires you to consider the information that you have available to you at the time of the evaluation and make a judgement as to whether the patient has progressed towards or moved away from the set goal. It also requires you to conclude whether the experience was right for them as an individual.

When carrying out final evaluation the nurse considers the baseline, goal and recheck information on the date set during the planning stage and evaluates whether the goal has been achieved by the patient. In doing this they are evaluating the process and the outcome. In other words, has the care been effective in allowing the patient to achieve their goal? When the goals have not been achieved, the process does not end; you need to restart the problem-solving process of ASPIRE and repeat the stages until the need is addressed. When all of the goals have been met or when completing the discharge plan, it is the time to establish whether the set goals were realistic and relevant and whether the prescribed care was appropriate in terms of meeting the goals. Issues of documentation and record keeping in relation to the patient's progress should be considered, along with choice of model so that an accurate, comprehensive evaluation can be made of how effective the approach has been. This means that the episode of care has been evaluated in terms of not only outcome but also the patient experience. In a sense it provides an audit trail of who did what and why they did it, so the care and experience is transparent for all to see and monitor.

When we outlined the skill of analysis in the assessment and systematic nursing diagnosis stage, we suggested that it involved taking very complex information, breaking it down into its individual parts, examining the parts and then reaching a considered conclusion. Ongoing and final evaluation require a practitioner to have the ability to critically analyse. This is because they involve taking the information from the baseline, goal and recheck stage and considering these separately, then comparing and contrasting the details to establish differences and similarities, and finally making a considered conclusion or evaluation as to whether the goal has been achieved.

Evaluating the *progress and process* in ongoing evaluation and *process and outcome* in final evaluation, is a complex skill that requires a sound knowledge base and the ability to critically analyse. It is for this reason that the recheck stage – monitoring, describing and documenting the current condition – can be conducted by a patient, relative, student nurse or care assistant. However, ongoing and final evaluation needs to be conducted by a qualified nurse or student nurse with supervision.

Figure 2.2 summarises the different elements of recheck and evaluation and what you try to ascertain at each step.

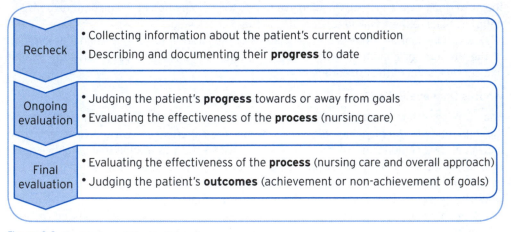

Figure 2.2 Recheck and Evaluation

WHAT HAVE YOU LEARNT SO FAR?

+ Evaluation is the final stage of ASPIRE.

+ You cannot make an informed decision during the evaluation stage without the use of a baseline.

+ The patient's behaviours/activities and personal accounts of their experiences become the focus for the decision making.

+ Ongoing evaluation decides whether the problem is getting better or getting worse by considering the progress and the process.

+ Final evaluation is to see whether the patient has achieved the set goal on the agreed date but also the patient experience.

+ Baselines, goals and recheck information are used to help the registered nurse to make the evaluation.

+ When expected outcomes do not take place, the cyclical process of ASPIRE is repeated.

+ Even if goals have been achieved, it is important to ask whether achieving the goal has solved or alleviated the problem, whether the goals were too easy, and whether there was an awareness of potential needs.

+ In a sense evaluation provides an audit trail of who did what and why they did it, so the care and experience is transparent for all to see and monitor.

+ Evaluation is a complex skill that requires a sound knowledge base and ability to analyse critically.

+ Ongoing and final evaluation need to be carried out by a registered nurse or student nurse under supervision.

Conclusion

It is important to remember that although the stages of ASPIRE have been described as separate steps they are interrelated and interdependent. Each stage offers information that leads to and directs the next stage. It cannot be emphasised too much how crucial it is to make sure that the process is based on the sound foundation of a good assessment. In a good assessment all the information for identifying the needs, planning, implementing and evaluating the care should be present in the description. Each stage will prove easier if the assessment has been conducted in a holistic, comprehensive way.

Further reading

As we have already discussed, the originators of the idea of a problem-solving approach to nursing care were Yura and Walsh in the 1960s. If you want to read more about this, then a later edition of their book is:

Yura H, Walsh M (1988) *The Nursing Process,* 5th ed. Norwalk, CT: Appleton & Lange.

There are many books out there which guide you through a problem-solving approach to patient care. Essentially, this it what we will be doing in the second half of this book, but if you want to look elsewhere, then another useful text is:

Carpenito-Moyet L (2005) *Understanding the Nursing Process: Concept Mapping and Care Planning for Students.* Philadelphia: Lippincott, Williams & Wilkins.

Chapter 3
Models of nursing and the Activities of Living Model

Why this chapter matters

If you've read Chapter 2, you will now be familiar with the problem-solving approach to care. This will help you when you next encounter a patient, because you will have an understanding of how the process of devising and delivering care should be structured. Unfortunately, the problem-solving approach to care isn't enough on its own, as it leaves many questions unanswered. For example, what questions do you need to ask the patient during the assessment stage? How would you recognise that a patient has a problem? What sort of interventions would you carry out as a nurse? How will you know if your interventions have been successful? These are all crucial questions, and they are not really answered by just referring to a problem-solving approach to care such as the nursing process or the adapted version – ASPIRE – that we looked at in the last chapter.

To make effective use of the problem-solving approach you need the help of something else – a model of nursing. Models of nursing can do much more than simply tell you what questions to ask during an assessment; they offer you a range of beliefs and values to guide you through the stages of the problem-solving process and offer you directions as to what is relevant and important during the stages. They are like a satellite navigation system, in the sense that they offer directions and guidance during the journey through the process of care planning and delivery, prompting you to take the right pathway.

This chapter will give you a brief introduction to nursing models and provide a more detailed look at one of the best known examples – the Activities of Living Model by Roper, Logan and Tierney (2000). It is not possible to do justice to the breadth of knowledge that each of the nursing models has to offer in the next three chapters; therefore, we suggest that you read the specific authors' accounts for a more in-depth understanding once you have mastered the basics.

By the end of this chapter you will be able to:

+ describe to a colleague what a model of nursing is;
+ talk about the main characteristics of the Activities of Living Model;
+ identify the possible strengths and limitations of the Activities of Living Model.

What is a model of nursing?

When attempting to define models of nursing, most books compare them to physical models, such as a model aeroplane. This is a good place to start, as there are usually two things that you expect with any model: first, models are made up of different parts; second, once the different parts are put together, they look like the real thing. Models of nursing are much the same. They are made up of different parts and, when put together, they will tell you what nursing is all about. In theory, if you understand a nursing model, then you have a picture of what nurses are and what nurses do. Models give direction to the nurse about the patients and their needs and define nursing roles derived from the views, beliefs and values about people, health, the environment and nursing. By doing so, models of nursing are intended to give the profession greater status and clarify exactly what nurses do as opposed to the roles of other members of the multidisciplinary team (such as doctors, pharmacists and physiotherapists).

At this point, many of the books start to discuss nursing theory and things called paradigms. We're not going to do this, not because we think that the material has nothing to offer, but because we don't want you to get bogged down by the theory and philosophical arguments at this point. We feel that it is more useful to outline the idea of a nursing model and demonstrate how this directs the nursing process; this way you can grasp the principles and start the process of learning how to use this framework to create effective, safe care plans. We've put some suggestions for further reading at the end of the chapter if you want to pursue these subjects further. First, have a go at Activity 3.1.

Activity 3.1

How many models of nursing have you heard of? Write down the authors of each and the things that you remember about them.

WHAT HAVE YOU LEARNT SO FAR?

+ Models of nursing try to describe what nurses are and what nurses do.
+ Models of nursing offer direction to the nurse about the patients and their needs, and define nursing roles derived from the views, beliefs and values about people, health, the environment and nursing.

Why do we need models?

It is worth clearing up a fairly major point at this stage. You will have noticed that we have made lots of reference to models of nursing – suggesting that there is more than one. The truth is there are lots; many are research-based, developed over years and published, but others are informal, evolved over time in response to changes in observed practice and shared by word of mouth. We plan to explore three published models in this book. One question that you might be asking is Why do we need so many models – doesn't one model fit all? The answer is 'no', partly because patients are individuals with complex, holistic needs, but also because nursing is a very broad term that embraces all the fields of nursing practice – mental health, child, adult and learning disability. Even within one field of nursing, the focus of the work can vary immensely – for example, in adult nursing, gynaecology compared with coronary care, or acute hospital care compared with community care. Whilst all nurses share a similar focus and approach, their roles and responsibilities differ. In the same way, nursing models share an interest in the topics that they consider – people, their environment, their health status and nursing goals – but their focus can differ. Consequently, it is important to find the right model for the right patient, which is why it is so useful to have a selection to choose from. Choosing a model that everyone in the nursing team can use leads to several advantages. In particular, models deliver consistency and continuity in the care to be delivered, because everyone will be working with the same underpinning philosophy when deciding and delivering the care. As a consequence of this there should be less conflict within the team and the adopted philosophy can act as a major guide to decision and policy-making (Pearson *et al.* 2005).

WHAT HAVE YOU LEARNT SO FAR?

+ There are lots of different nursing models – some are formal and published in books and articles, whilst others are informal and shared by word of mouth.

+ Even though there are a variety of nursing models, they all share an interest in the topics that they consider – people, their environment, their health status and nursing goals. The difference between them is their focus of interest.

+ We need a variety of models because patients are individuals with complex needs and nursing is a broad term that embraces all the fields of nursing.

+ It is important to choose the right model for the right patient, and one which also best fits the working environment.

+ Having a model that everyone can share and identify with can lead to several advantages that will benefit the team and the patient.

How does the nursing model fit with a problem-solving approach to care?

It is important to recognise that there is a relationship between nursing models and the problem-solving approach. As mentioned previously, the nursing process gives structure to care delivery, whereas a model describes how it should actually be done (Walsh 1998).

This would seem to imply that you cannot have one without the other, because the process defines the stages that we should take, whilst the model tells us how we should be carrying out the stages. In other words, the model tells us what is important and relevant when devising and delivering individualised care. The challenge for the nursing team is to choose the right model for their clinical area: one that offers their nursing specialty the right guidance, but that also suits the needs of the patient. Sometimes a team may generate their own informal model based on a variety of nursing models by selecting the elements that best fit with their requirements: this is called an eclectic approach.

In a way, it could be said that nursing models are the tools of our trade. A joiner has a set of different screwdrivers in their toolbox to allow them to choose a special type of head for a particular job. This saves time and effort and ensures that an efficient, safe job is done. When the joiner becomes skilled at their craft, they often adapt their tools to suit their requirements, even if it is just to stir their tea. Similarly, we have a selection of nursing models to help us devise, deliver and monitor care and, once we become proficient and skilled in their use, we can be creative and adaptive or eclectic in our use of them.

WHAT HAVE YOU LEARNT SO FAR?

+ There is a relationship between nursing models and the problem-solving approach – the process defines the stages we should take, whilst a model describes how we should carry out the stages.

+ Nursing teams may generate their own informal model based on a variety of nursing models by selecting the elements that best fit with their requirements, known as an eclectic approach.

For the rest of the book, we're going to concentrate on three well-known models of nursing. These are the Activities of Living Model, by Roper, Logan and Tierney – which the rest of this chapter is devoted to – Orem's Self-Care Model of Nursing, and the Neuman Systems Model of Nursing. The fact that we're looking at these three doesn't in any way mean that these are the 'best' of the models available. However, they are fairly well known in clinical practice and we think they provide a good indication of the range of ideas in different models.

Roper, Logan and Tierney's Activities of Living Model

Roper, Logan and Tierney (we're going to shorten the names of this trio of nurse theorists to RLT for the remainder of the book) offer a representation of nursing that considers the living person as a whole entity rather than a medical label or 'the appendix in bed four'. They wanted to move away from a disease-based approach to care, one that looks at the illness and managing the signs and symptoms, to an approach that recognises the holistic needs of the individual. They stress the importance of cultural, environmental and economic factors affecting both health and well-being and encourage a nursing role in preventing, alleviating or coping with illness. Important ideas that can be found within the model are:

+ individuality;
+ the activities of living;
+ a dependence–independence continuum;
+ the progression of a person along a lifespan continuum;
+ influencing factors.

Individuality

This is the idea that every person is an individual. Whilst they may share things in common with others, they are unique in the way they carry out their everyday lives. It then follows that the individual should be central to all stages of a problem-solving approach to care. Particular attention needs to be given over to their individual way of carrying out their everyday activities, and involvement in deciding what their goals are and how they will achieve them should be encouraged wherever possible.

Activities of living

RLT (2000) identify 12 activities of living (see Exhibit 3.1). Each activity represents a particular type of behaviour that all of us carry out on a day-to-day basis whilst interacting with each other and our environment. Some of the activities of living are essential to keeping us alive, whilst others enhance our quality of life and as such are not seen as essential. Because the individual is best understood in terms of the activities that they can and cannot carry out, the 12 activities offer a way of identifying the common nursing requirements shared by all patients. The activities of living are meant to represent the common elements of everyday living that

1. Maintaining a safe environment
2. Communicating
3. Breathing
4. Eating and drinking
5. Eliminating
6. Personal cleansing and dressing
7. Controlling body temperature
8. Working and playing
9. Mobilising
10. Sleeping
11. Expressing sexuality
12. Dying

Roper, Logan and Tierney (2000)

Exhibit 3.1 The 12 activities of living

ensure our survival and quality of life. Given that, do 12 activities really reflect the complex nature of living? If you interpret them in a very narrow way, and use them as a 'checklist' when assessing a patient, then the list doesn't cover everything. For example, where would you put the patient's descriptions of their pain, or acknowledge their religious and spiritual beliefs? However, if you use them as a way of categorising the detailed information gained from a comprehensive assessment and view them as the model intends, then they do address our daily activities of living in a holistic manner. First, it is important to remember that the activities do not exist as separate entities, because each one is interrelated to the other 11. This will become obvious when you start exploring the case studies in the forthcoming chapters and witness how illness and health can affect a patient's independence. Secondly, the categories are meant to represent the activity in its broadest sense; to help illustrate this, it may prove useful to consider each one in turn and explore what they represent.

We need to make it very clear at this point that the following descriptions are not an exhaustive account of what should go under each of the headings. This would be almost impossible because patients are individuals and will always have some needs that are unexpected and also because the categories are not meant to be used as a checklist. Some of the factors and details included in the categories would not be appropriate or relevant to the care of every patient; you are not expected to explore all the suggestions or even all the categories. However, they can act as a framework for the assessment process by offering direction for the discussion between you and the patient and by providing a way of categorising the information you found out about the person and their ability to perform the activity. How you conduct the assessment using the activities of living model will be discussed later, in Chapter 8, but it is worth remembering that the information documented under the headings should include the answers to the following questions:

+ What can you normally do?
+ What can you do now?
+ Is there a change or difference?
+ What is causing the change or difference?
+ What are you doing about it?
+ What is anyone else doing about it?
+ How do you deal with the problem now or in the past?

Maintaining a safe environment

Maintaining a safe environment aims to protect the individual from harm of any sort, so potentially this heading could encompass just about anything that the patient is in contact with that may cause harm or illness. There are two types of environment that need to be considered: external and internal. The external environment is the space outside of us, from the immediate space just outside your body, to the world at large. The internal environment, not surprisingly, describes the space within each of us.

Maintaining a safe external environment covers a whole host of issues, such as hand washing and cross-infection, housing conditions, environmental pollution, poverty and social deprivation, and global influences such as world economy, war and the effects of global warming. Maintaining a safe internal environment is concerned with **homeostasis** within the individual; therefore hormone and chemical imbalances, bleeding, pain, disruptions to vital signs or any of the systems can be included in this category. It also includes the disruptions that occur as a result of personal lifestyle choices and psychological factors such as depression, anxiety, confusion and lack of knowledge.

Communicating

This activity refers to the act of communication in all its forms. Information about the patient's ability to interact with others and their ability to use verbal, non-verbal communication and listening skills is recorded under this heading. Factors that disrupt communication such as loss of any of the senses, shyness, autism, arguments, and falling out with friends and relatives need to be considered. Acknowledging alternative ways of communicating such as lip reading, sign language, therapeutic touch, reading and writing, computers or picture boards is also relevant.

Breathing

Being able to carry out the activity of breathing relies upon a fully functioning cardiovascular and respiratory system. Measurements that indicate lung function and breathing capacity can be included here – respiration (depth, rate, noise), colour of skin and **mucous membranes** and **peak flow** – but also information that relates to oxygen saturation, blood gases, use of **accessory muscles of respiration** and haemoglobin levels. Factors that influence breathing such as infection, disorders and illness, smoking, pollution, anxiety and strategies that help with breathing such as positioning when sleeping, breathing exercises, oxygen therapy and fitness levels need to be noted. If a cough is present, a full description, including the type and presence of mucus or discharge, could be recorded here.

Eating and drinking

Eating and drinking relies on the ability to bite, chew, swallow and digest. Nutritional knowledge, ability to cook and shop, likes, dislikes and finances will determine your choice of food

Homeostasis is a state in which the body's internal environment remains constant.

Mucous membranes are thin sheets of tissue that line different parts of the body such as the inside of the mouth.

Peak flow is the maximum rate of air flow achieved when breathing out.

Accessory muscles of respiration are muscles in the abdomen, back and neck that may help with breathing during exercise or illness.

and drink. Equally, cultural differences, religious beliefs and restrictions, attitudes towards food and drink and body image will all influence this activity. These may need to be explored and recorded as well as the patient's nutritional state, hydration level, weight, eating patterns, cholesterol levels and metabolic or absorption disorders.

Eliminating

Eliminating refers to the excretion of waste products such as urine and faeces, so it is not surprising that this activity concentrates on describing how patients maintain and perform their normal bladder and bowel function. Difficulties and treatments or coping strategies are also noted. However, restricting this activity to urine and faeces would produce a rather narrow exploration, so assessment may need to include a broader interpretation and include things such as excretion of excess carbon dioxide in breath, bile salts in the skin, vomit, pus and discharge from wounds, mucus from the nose and throat, vaginal discharge and water and toxins in sweat.

Personal cleansing and dressing

This activity does include washing and bathing habits but it also extends to the maintenance of hair, nails and teeth and mouth care. Dress code and rituals, some of which may be related to religious and spiritual beliefs, or even personality and individual differences, need to be included in here.

Controlling body temperature

Controlling body temperature relates to the activities that the patient carries out to keep their internal and external temperature at a comfortable level. These include temperature increase, sweating, flushing, shivering, putting extra clothes on or taking them off, using fans, turning on the central heating and eating hot or cold foods and drink. Measurements of core temperature could be recorded here, but also the localised temperature changes that occur to the skin and tissues indicating infection; skin that becomes warm to the touch and red or inflamed can also be noted here.

Working and playing

Working refers to paid employment but also unpaid activities that the individual engages in, such as housework, DIY and gardening. Playing refers to the recreational activities that individuals carry out in order to relax, unwind and have fun; this might include going to the cinema, visiting the pub, dancing or going to the gym.

Mobilising

Mobilising refers to movement in terms of walking, running and bending – activities that involve the large muscles, ligaments, tendons and skeletal system – but it also relates to the fine motor skills involved in manual dexterity, facial expressions, mannerisms, tics and non-verbal communication. Factors that disrupt these activities such as pain, arthritis, paralysis, injury and depression need to be noted, as well as the individual ways of carrying out the movements. Potential problems such as pressure ulcers that can arise from enforced bed rest and details of skin integrity can be recorded in this category.

Sleeping

The ability to sleep and relax needs to be considered in this category. The quality of sleep and identification of the factors that stop us sleeping such as acid reflux, night sweats, a noisy ward environment, fears, worries, pain, restrictions imposed by infusion devices, catheters and drains need to be documented. Whether a patient engages in **rapid eye movement (REM) sleep** or has nightmares should be noted, because fitful sleep depletes the patient's ability to think and will cause disruptions to the immune system. Sleeping too much or irregular sleep patterns such as taking daytime naps need to be considered, as well as routines that encourage the patient to sleep.

Expressing sexuality

Expressing sexuality is more than sexual function and activity. This category could include all the information that relates to establishing and maintaining sexual health; this would include knowledge and understanding of reproduction, contraception and safe sex, puberty, menstruation and menopause. Feeling comfortable with your sexual identity, being able to express your sexuality in the way you dress and your personal appearance (such as make-up, hairstyle and perfume) are included in this activity. Equally important is the consideration of the roles and responsibilities we adopt that are related to expressing our sexuality: mother, father, wife, boyfriend, homemaker, breadwinner etc.

Dying

This activity is concerned with all aspects related to the act of dying: thoughts, fears, concerns, treatments, general beliefs, religious beliefs, rituals, requests and personal wishes. In other words, this is all the information that would help an individual carry out this activity in comfort and with respect and dignity. However, consideration of this activity is not limited to patients with a life-threatening illness or terminal diagnosis. Exploration may need to occur with a patient having surgery or awaiting the results of an investigation. In the case of Suzy Clarke (see scenario in Appendix A) this is relevant because she fears she is going to die. It is also true to say that patients experiencing grief, loss or deprivation as a result of losing someone or something – a loved one, a limb, a breast, a role or responsibility – may need to have this activity explored.

Lastly it should be noted that to die successfully, you have to live successfully; it is for this reason that spiritual issues and concerns could be considered under this heading. How does the patient appraise their life? Is it a full, content existence or a miserable, empty lonely experience? What are their spiritual and/or religious beliefs? Do they bring comfort or are they looking for help, guidance and direction? The answers to these questions can be recorded under this heading.

Now look at Activity 3.2.

Activity 3.2

Can you identify which of the activities are essential for life maintenance and which enhance the quality of life? Are there any that fall into both categories?

Rapid eye movement (REM) sleep is the period of sleep when dreaming occurs.

RLT argue that of the 12 activities of living, certain activities are seen as biologically determined whilst others are decided by the individual's social and cultural experiences. What does this mean?

Activities that are biologically determined are behaviours that have developed because of genetic inheritance and biological influences. This suggests that your ability to carry out some of the activities of living has something to do with your ancestors and how your body and mind have developed over time as a consequence of biological influences such as genes, hormones, bodily chemicals and processes and interaction with the external environment. The 'environmental influence' is related to how environmental factors (diet, drugs, immediate surroundings, accidents etc.) affect biological development and physiological processes rather than how family, society, experience and learning shape behaviour and mental processes.

Examples of biologically determined behaviours are the ability to breathe and walk. Both of these behaviours are dependent on your genetic inheritance and a fully functioning biological system. Some of these biological influences seem very obvious: for example, you need to be born with fully functioning lungs to take your first breath and strong legs to walk. What might not be so obvious is that the force or volume of your breath, as measured by your peak flow and the age at which you learn to walk, are also a result of biology, because both of these activities are determined by your genes. Biologically determined behaviours can be influenced by the environment – both internal and external and it is easy to see how environmental factors such as nutrition, pollution, housing conditions and the opportunity to practise walking can influence the activity of breathing and walking.

Socially and culturally determined refers to the way in which your cultural and social circumstances have influenced the activities of living. The values, beliefs and norms of the community that you grow up in will influence your ability and the way that you carry out the activities of living. Examples of this would be what, how and when you eat and drink, how you go about your personal cleansing and what you choose to wear, how you communicate, and rituals and practices around death and dying, parenting and expressing sexuality.

In summary the ways in which you go about your activities of living are a result of biological influences and the community that you grow up and live in. It is these factors that create the individual and define the uniqueness in which they go about their everyday activities. Now consider Activity 3.3.

Activity 3.3

Think about the way in which you carry out the 12 activities of living. List those that are biologically determined and those that are socially and culturally determined. Take a look at your list. It is unique to you because this is what makes you who you are and ensures that you are very different from others around you.

Dependence–independence continuum

By now it should be clear that people differ in the way that they engage in the 12 activities as discussed. What adds to the individuality of the way a person carries out the activities is how independent or dependent they are, or what they can and cannot do for themselves. RLT introduce the idea of a dependence–independence continuum, a scale that identifies where the individual is generally, in terms of carrying out the activity of living.

The following influence the individual's general position on the continuum:

+ maturity;
+ social and economic circumstances;
+ cultural background.

Maturity

Maturity or age will influence where an individual falls on the dependence–independence contin-uum, or in other words what they can or cannot do for themselves. It is easy to see that a baby is more dependent than an adult in communicating, eating and drinking and personal cleansing and dressing. Equally, movement along the continuum towards dependence may occur as you get older, but not always. Being young doesn't necessarily make you less independent and older more so; a baby may be considered more independent than an adult who smokes in terms of carrying out the activity of breathing. Therefore, it is important to consider all the activities one by one in terms of the individual's general position on the continuum, because each activity may have a different level of independence. One last thing to remember is that an individual's posi-tion is not static and can change over a relatively short period of time.

Social and economic circumstances

Social and economic circumstances can influence the individual's position on the continuum; think about the activities of maintaining a safe environment, eating and drinking and work-ing and playing. If you are a single parent living on benefits on a sprawling housing estate on the city outskirts, your social and economic circumstances could influence whether you can afford the bus fare to attend a well-person clinic, what and when you eat and whether you can go to the cinema to unwind.

Cultural background

Equally, cultural background can influence your position on the continuum. The way that you were brought up, and the values, beliefs and norms that you were exposed to will influence what you are willing and able to do for yourself and how you carry out your everyday behaviours.

The three factors above will dictate how independent or dependent you are in relation to the activities of living, but people may not involve themselves in certain activities because of personal choice or a lack of social and economic opportunity. It may be, for example, that you don't want to get dressed or wash your hair today because you just feel like relaxing in front of the television or that you believe that washing every day is unnecessary and choose to take a bath every week instead. Equally, you may choose not to eat certain foods or decide to eat a diet of snacks and ready meals that you don't have to prepare. Social and economic circumstances can influence controlling body temperature and eating and drink-ing. As a student trying to live on a limited budget, your circumstances will influence whether you turn up the central heating or what you can afford to eat. Yet the social opportunity of living in a community with lots of friends would probably mean that you could engage in the activity of communicating very well, but maybe not sleeping for as many hours as you would like. Work through Activity 3.4.

Activity 3.4

Think about the following activities of living: eating and drinking, personal cleansing and dressing, working and playing and expressing sexuality. Where are you on the dependence–independence continuum (what you can and cannot do) in relation to carrying out these activities?

Identify how maturity, social and economic circumstances and cultural background decide your general position. Do personal choice and lack of social and economic opportunity mean that you have to review your usual position?

The progression of a person along a lifespan continuum

Roper, Logan and Tierney believe that the individual passes through eight developmental stages from conception to death. Different needs will arise as the individual reaches each of the stages, and changes in age may cause movement up or down the continuum, influencing what the individual can or cannot do. The stages are:

+ infancy (conception to 5 years);
+ childhood (6–12 years);
+ adolescence (13–18 years);
+ early adulthood (19–30 years);
+ middle years (31–45 years);
+ late adulthood (46–65 years);
+ old age (66 years and above).

It is necessary to acknowledge that developmental needs don't just refer to the demands that arise from the physical changes that accompany maturity. It is equally important to consider the psychological and sociocultural needs that arise as the individual progresses along the lifespan continuum. There are various theorists that can offer you an insight and understanding of the developmental process and the psychological and sociocultural needs that occur as we develop from the cradle to the grave. One common theme running through many of the developmental theories is that each stage along the lifespan continuum offers different physical, psychological and sociocultural challenges that the individual must undertake. Linking this to the model, it suggests that experiences associated with the developmental stages (infancy, childhood, adolescence, puberty, menopause, death) and experiences from life events (going to school, forming relationships, marriage, divorce, unemployment, bereavement) will result in specific developmental needs because they affect the way in which we carry out the activities of living. Where the patient is on the lifespan continuum needs to be identified and considered, as it can have a real impact on how the patient carries out the activities of living.

Influencing factors

We have talked about the circumstances that can influence an individual's general position on the dependence–independence continuum, but what are the factors that can result in movement along the continuum to a point at which the individual is likely to require nursing intervention? Roper, Logan and Tierney suggest that it is the influencing factors that can cause movement along the continuum, from relative independence to relative dependence for one or more of the 12 activities of living. The factors fall into five categories:

+ Biological – accidents, infections, disease, disability, but also the individual's anatomical structure and physical performance, which is determined by genetic and biological influences.
+ Sociocultural – religious beliefs, cultural norms, values, class, religion and gender, but also changes in social circumstances can all influence the carrying out of the activities and the development of the individual.
+ Psychological – emotional state, mood, temperament, motivation, intelligence, perception, stress, anxiety, fear, knowledge base as well as cognitive functioning. The way you think and process can be influenced by drugs, alcohol and lack of sleep. All of these psychological factors can impact on the way an activity is carried out by the individual.
+ Environmental – family and housing conditions, neighbourhood, national and global environments.
+ Politicoeconomic – resources and conditions that are dictated and governed by the relevant society's laws, economy and social policies. In turn, these will influence poverty levels and benefit systems, healthcare provision and education systems.

Have a go at Activity 3.5.

Activity 3.5

Consider the scenario for Suzy Clarke (see Appendix A). Can you identify the influencing factors that are affecting Suzy's position on the dependence–independence continuum? List the influencing factors and identify what activities they are affecting.

Your examples for Activity 3.5 may have included the following:

+ Physical – **anaemia** is influencing the activities of maintaining a safe environment, breathing, working and playing and mobilising.
+ Sociocultural – Suzy's standards of cleanliness and tidiness are influencing the activities of maintaining a safe environment, communicating and working and playing with her flatmates.

Anaemia is low levels of haemoglobin in the blood. It can cause tiredness, breathlessness and dizziness.

+ Psychological – panic attacks are influencing the activities of maintaining a safe environment, breathing, working and playing, mobilising, sleeping and dying.
+ Environmental – poor housing conditions are affecting the activities of maintaining a safe environment and controlling body temperature.
+ Politicoeconomic – living on a student bursary is influencing the activities of maintaining a safe environment, eating and drinking, personal cleansing and dressing, controlling body temperature and working and playing.

It is when there is movement along the dependence–independence continuum to the point that it influences what the individual can do for themselves that a problem is said to exist. In response to this movement, RLT suggest that there are three types of activity (behaviour) in which the nurse and patient can participate in order to address the problem:

+ Preventing behaviours – actions that reduce health risks and encourage health behaviours, such as bathing to prevent infections, changing position in bed to prevent a deep vein thrombosis, immunisation to prevent illness and disease and exercise to reduce the risk of coronary heart disease later in life.
+ Comforting behaviours – activities that make a person feel better. This will include physical behaviours such as arranging pillows and offering warm drinks, but also psychological and social behaviours. These would include reassuring someone, encouraging the use of coping strategies to deal with a stressful situation, the use of appropriate touch, talking and listening to someone and arranging for a social worker to offer advice on legal and social entitlements.
+ Seeking behaviours – activities that help gain knowledge or information that may benefit the patient's health such as going to the GP, asking the pharmacist or NHS Direct for advice, looking on the Internet and reading leaflets, journals and books.

What these three behaviours have in common is that they all strive to keep the patient well or help them to return to their optimum level of health and well-being. It is therefore important to make sure that the delivery of care is seen to be based around these activities and involve actions that acquire, maintain and restore independence in relation to the 12 activities of living.
Now try Activity 3.6.

Activity 3.6

Think about Suzy Clarke from Appendix A. Can you identify the actions that you as the nurse and Suzy as the patient need to participate in to deal with the problems of panic attacks? List them under the headings of preventing, seeking and comforting behaviours.

Strengths of the model

The RLT Model of Nursing is one of the most commonly used within the United Kingdom (Tierney 1998). For this reason, it is generally well known and many nurses are comfortable using it.

There are a number of reasons for its popularity. First, it was written by British nurses, so much of the language related to the model is familiar to those in the UK. In addition, the concepts discussed within the model are fairly simple and straightforward and offer an algorithmic format and structure that reassures nurses, particularly novice student nurses (Pudner 2005). In comparison – as we will discuss in Chapters 4 and 5 – some of the American nursing models can contain rather complex and 'flowery' language and include reference to some difficult theoretical concepts.

Equally, using assessment tools can duplicate and compartmentalise the information, which in turn can lead to uncoordinated, fragmented care. RLT frame the information and allow the practitioner to collate the findings, allowing them to see the impact of the changes on all 12 activities of living.

One further characteristic of the RLT model is that it recognises that medicine and nursing cannot be considered separately. Whereas doctors may be primarily concerned with curing disease and nurses with helping patients cope with the effects of disease, these two broad aims are closely linked. In fact, the commonalities that arise can facilitate multidisciplinary working and shared understanding (Humphries and Heans 2004). By acknowledging this, the RLT model is often seen as reflecting the reality of modern healthcare.

Limitations of the model

Although the RLT model is popular amongst many UK nurses, it does have a number of critics. The links to medical care that are addressed above have led to accusations of the model being too medically and hospital-oriented.

In addition, some critics claim that the model is oversimplified and concentrates on dealing with biological factors at the cost of other, equally important factors (Tierney 1998). After all, the activities of living are all physical, with the emphasis on identifying if the patient can carry out the tasks. Many of these criticisms do seem a little unfair. For example, Walsh (1998) suggests that the model has no psychological or social dimension, despite the presence of the influencing factors within the model itself. Walsh describes the RLT assessment as a 'checklist', and uses this as a basis for criticising the simplicity of the model. Some practitioners may not include information about their patients' pain and religious or spiritual beliefs if they cannot decide what category to use, or may add extra headings, making the assessment and documentation process even longer than is necessary. However, as we've explored above, the 12 activities of living should never be used as a checklist. Used properly, they will provide a detailed and holistic assessment, something that is not always acknowledged by critics.

Now consider Activity 3.7.

Activity 3.7

Think about your own experiences of using the RLT model. What do you like about the model, and what do you think the weaknesses are?

Conclusion

This chapter has provided an introduction to nursing models in general, and the RLT model in particular. We've explored how nursing models start to fill in some of the gaps left by the nursing process, and actually tell you how to assess, diagnose, plan, implement and evaluate. The RLT model is the most commonly used in the UK, and we've begun to look at the values that underpin it. It is undoubtedly one of the simplest models to use. Although this might leave it open for criticism, it also makes it ideal for student or newly qualified nurses to use. The second section of the book will actually show you how to put the RLT model (in addition to others) into practice.

Further reading

If you want to read more about nursing theories, concepts and paradigms, then Pearson, Vaughan and Fitzgerald provide an interesting account in Chapter 4, 'The basis of models', in:

Pearson A, Vaughan B, Fitzgerald M (2005) *Nursing Models for Practice* 3rd ed. Edinburgh: Butterworth Heinemann.

If you want to read more about developmental theories, then we would recommend:

Bee H, Boyd D (2006) *The Developing Child,* 11th ed. New York: HarperCollins.

In terms of specific models, a more detailed account can always be found in the text written by the originators of the model themselves. In the case of the Activities of Living Model, the latest edition of this is:

Roper N, Logan W, Tierney A (2000) *The Roper Logan Tierney Model of Nursing*. Edinburgh: Churchill Livingstone.

There is also a textbook devoted to the application of the Activities of Living Model, which is presented in a very readable manner:

Holland K, Jenkins J, Solomon J, Whittam S (2008) *Applying the Roper–Logan–Tierney Model in Practice*, 2nd ed. Edinburgh: Churchill Livingstone.

Chapter 4
Orem's Self-Care Model of Nursing

Why this chapter matters

In the last chapter, we gave you an introduction to nursing models generally, and the Activities of Living Model specifically. As we highlighted, there are many nursing models in existence, all with a slightly different view of people, health, the environment and nursing.

Looking at the Activities of Living Model has outlined just one set of ideas, but it is important to have different viewpoints when planning care for your patients. To that end, this chapter looks at another very popular model of nursing – Orem's Self-Care Model.

By the end of the chapter, you will be able to:

+ identify the main characteristics of Orem's Self-Care Model;
+ identify the possible strengths and limitations of the Self-Care Model.

Introduction to the model

Orem's model is a holistic model, in that the person is considered as a whole, rather than as separate systems (for example, nervous, skeletal, urinary) or parts of the body (for example, nursing a leg ulcer). A holistic model guides the user in considering the physical, psychological, social and spiritual aspects of a person's life. There should not be undue emphasis placed on one aspect, for example just considering physical factors. 'Holism can be defined as recognition that all dimensions of the individual – physical, social, psychological and spiritual – are attended to with equal importance' (McSherry, 2007). Dorothea Orem was American (she died in 2007 at the age of 92) and originally wrote this model for academic use; as a result of this, the language can be difficult to understand, but try not to be put off as we will be explaining the terms that she used. It is important to understand that although it is called the self-care model, its use should not be restricted to people who can look after themselves. This model can be used for all types of patients, ranging from those who rely on others for all of their care (for example, a patient in an intensive care unit) to patients who just require a little bit of help (a patient requiring some health advice). By the end of this chapter, you will be able to see how versatile it is in meeting different client groups' needs.

The important ideas underlying the model are:

+ self-care/self-care agency;
+ universal self-care requisites (USCRs);
+ developmental self-care requisites (DSCRs);
+ health deviation self-care requisites (HDSCRs);
+ helping methods and the nursing systems.

Self-care/self-care agency

Orem (2001) believed that both maturing and mature adults have the capacity and capability to regulate their own functioning and development. She refers to this as 'self-care agency' and the person looking after themselves as the 'self-care agent'. Put simply, adults, when healthy, want to and can look after themselves; they have the ability to be self-caring. However, to do this they have to possess the skills, knowledge, desire (motivation) and range of behaviours to carry out the activities essential to live a healthy life. Orem argued that people have the motivation and the potential to acquire the relevant skills, knowledge, desire and behaviour in them to be self-caring and also to look after people who depend upon them for care, for example their children or elderly relatives or an ill partner; she referred to this as 'dependent care'.

When a person becomes unwell, is injured, or has a problem with their development, they may not have the skill, knowledge, desire or behaviour to cope with looking after themselves. This means there is a difference in what they are able to do and what they need to do for themselves. Orem called this a 'self-care deficit', and it can be seen as equivalent to what Roper, Logan and Tierney (discussed in the last chapter) would refer to as a problem. The illness, injury and/or development needs that cause the self-care deficit or problem are referred to as the therapeutic self-care demand, or just the 'self-care demand'.

When a self-care demand occurs and other members of the family or friends cannot address the deficit or problem, then nursing care is needed. Orem referred to the input from nurses as 'nursing agency'. According to Orem the goal of nursing addresses the deficit by either increasing the patient's capacity to meet the demand or reducing the demand upon the patient. An example of raising the patient's capacity may be teaching them some new knowledge or skill. Alternatively, reducing the demand upon the patient could involve advising rest when the patient has an infection, thereby reducing the demands on the body for food, fluid and oxygen. Consider Practice example 4.1.

Practice example 4.1

Evelyn, a 72-year old woman, develops diabetes mellitus for which she will require daily insulin injections. If she can master the skill of giving her own injections (increase her capacity), then she will remain self-caring. If, however, she is unable to develop the skill and there is no one to do this for her, she will have a self-care deficit – a gap in her ability to look after herself. This means that she will require a nurse to give her injections. Evelyn is reliant on the nurse giving the injections to her and so the nurse is said to be providing nursing agency. If there was a relative or friend of Evelyn's that could give the injections, then this would be referred to as providing dependent care and they would be the dependent-care agent.

WHAT HAVE YOU LEARNT SO FAR?

+ The self-care agent is the person looking after themselves.
+ Self-care agency is the ability to look after yourself.
+ Individuals have to have the appropriate skills, knowledge, motivation and range of behaviours to look after themselves.
+ Dependent care is when a person gives care to another person.
+ A self-care deficit occurs when the person cannot maintain self-care due to a self-care demand.
+ A self-care demand can occur as a result of illness, injury and/or development needs.
+ Nursing agency refers to the input of nurses to help a patient with their care.

Universal self-care requisites (USCRs)

Orem believed that, in order to remain healthy, there are eight basic needs that have to be met; she calls these the universal self-care requisites (USCRs). Let's break the term down and explore what is meant by it. A requisite is a requirement or need; universal refers to the fact that it is something that everyone has in common. We have already established that self-care refers to the care that people engage in to live a healthy life, so universal self-care requisites are needs that have to be fulfilled by everyone to live a healthy life. Have a look at Activity 4.1.

Activity 4.1

Can you think what the universal self-care requisites are? It might help you, when you make your list, to think about what human beings need in order to remain healthy and not just to live or survive. It will help if you think back to Roper, Logan and Tierney's activities of living.

Your list from Activity 4.1 will probably have included some of the eight USCRs that Orem identified (see Exhibit 4.1), but you may have used different words. Some of the words and phrases Orem used may seem complicated, but we will be exploring their meaning and relevance to nursing using terms that you will be able to understand.

1. Sufficient intake of air
2. Sufficient intake of water
3. Sufficient intake of food
4. Satisfactory eliminative functions
5. Activity balanced with rest
6. Balance between solitude and social interaction
7. Prevention of hazards to human life, human functioning and human well-being
8. Promotion of human functioning and development within social groups in accordance with human potential, known human limitations and the desire for 'normalcy'

Exhibit 4.1 The universal self-care requisites

People will meet the eight USCRs in different ways according to their culture, ethnic origin, educational background, temperament, illness etc. It is important for nurses to accept that one person may meet their USCRs in a different way to others; it does not make it wrong, just different. Nurses need to ensure that any preconceived prejudices that they might hold do not interfere with how they care for people (NMC 2008). This is a similar idea to RLT's individuality in that, although people share commonalities, they are unique in the way they carry out their everyday lives. As with RLT's activities of living, Orem did not want the eight USCRs to be used as a checklist when assessing patients, but rather as a framework to help you to conduct a holistic assessment that considers physical, psychological, social and spiritual aspects of the person. With any model, a useful way of ensuring a comprehensive assessment is carried out, is to use the questions identified earlier when discussing ASPIRE in Chapter 2:

✚ What can you normally do?

✚ What can you do now?

✚ Is there a change or difference?

✚ What is causing the change or difference?

✚ What are you doing about it?

✚ What is anyone else doing about it?

✚ How did you deal with the problem in the past (if relevant)?

Let's explore what type of information could be categorised under each of the USCRs, following an assessment; this will help you to understand what Orem meant by each of the USCRs. The examples that we offer are not exhaustive, because each person will meet their USCRs in a way that is unique to them. It is important to remember that the USCRs are inter-related and that a self-care deficit in one may produce an effect in another; for example, if there is insufficient intake of air due to a chest infection, then the USCR of activity balanced with rest can be affected (a person may have to reduce their activity and rest more). How to conduct an assessment using Orem's model will be discussed in Chapter 8.

1. Sufficient intake of air

Having a sufficient intake of air relies upon a functioning cardiovascular and respiratory system. Measurements that indicate lung function, breathing and circulatory capacity can be included here – blood pressure, pulse (rate, rhythm, volume), respiration (depth, rate, noise), colour of skin and mucous membranes, peak flow – and also information that relates to oxygen saturation, blood gases, use of accessory muscles and haemoglobin levels. Factors that influence breathing such as infection, disorders and illness, smoking, pollution and anxiety and also strategies that help with breathing, such as positioning when sleeping, breathing exercises, oxygen therapy and levels of fitness need to be noted. If a cough is present a full description including the type, colour and amount of mucus or discharge could be recorded here.

2. and 3. Sufficient intake of water and sufficient intake of food (these two are often considered together)

Sufficient intake of water and sufficient intake of food rely on the ability to bite, chew, swallow and digest. Nutritional knowledge, ability to cook and shop, likes, dislikes and finances will determine your choice of food and drink. Equally, cultural differences, religious beliefs and restrictions, attitudes towards food and drink and body image will all influence this activity. These may need to be explored and recorded as well as the patient's nutritional state, hydration level, weight, eating patterns, cholesterol, metabolic disorders and allergies.

4. Satisfactory eliminative functions

Elimination refers to the excretion of waste products such as urine and faeces, so this USCR concentrates on describing how patients maintain and perform their normal bowel and bladder function. Difficulties and treatments or coping strategies are also noted. As with RLT's definition of elimination, we don't want to narrow this USCR simply to urine and faeces, so assessment may need to include a broader interpretation and include excretion of waste products through the skin or breathing, vomit, pus and discharge from wounds, vaginal discharge, water and toxins in sweat. Orem (2001) also identified hygiene-related care of both the body and the environment in order to maintain clean conditions. Therefore things to be included would be washing and bathing habits, maintenance of **perianal** hygiene, and care of hair, nails, teeth and mouth.

5. Activity balanced with rest

This does not just mean physical activity and resting, but also psychological activity. Activity refers to paid and unpaid employment and leisure activities such as engaging in sports, hobbies and holidays. Intellectual activity may include undertaking educational classes, playing chess, and engaging in puzzles and crosswords. Rest includes sleeping and restful activities. The quality of sleep and identification of the factors that stop us sleeping such as acid reflux, night sweats, a noisy environment, fears, worries, pain and restrictions imposed by infusion devices, catheters and drains need to be documented. Sleeping too much or irregular sleep patterns such as taking daytime naps need to be considered as well as routines that encourage the patient to sleep. Orem believed that each person must maintain a balance between activity and rest; for example, a person who sits in an office all day as their paid employment may need an active hobby, whereas a landscape gardener may require a less active hobby.

Perianal is the area around the anus.

Activity also refers specifically to movement in terms of walking, running and bending – activities that involve the large muscles, ligaments, tendons and skeletal system – but it also relates to the fine motor skills involved in manual dexterity, facial expressions, mannerisms, tics and non-verbal communication. Factors that disrupt these activities such as pain, arthritis, paralysis, injury and depression need to be noted as well as the individual ways of carrying out the movements. Potential problems such as pressure ulcers that can arise from enforced bed rest and details of skin integrity can be recorded in this self-care requisite.

6. Balance between solitude and social interaction

This refers to the need for some time on your own for reflection and to develop a sense of self, balanced with the need to develop bonds of affection and friendship and loving relationships, both in one-to-one relationships and in groups. It is about learning how to manage relationships with other individuals and social groups. Factors that could be considered are the type and number of social activities engaged in and the type and quality of individual and group relationships. Some people are happy with their own company and actively seek solitude; others do not like being alone and want company. This will vary from person to person, and so the balance between solitude and social interaction will be different for different individuals.

7. Prevention of hazards to human life, human functioning and human well-being

This requires the person to be aware of hazards (dangers) to their physical, psychological and social self. It is about protecting the individual from harm of any sort, so potentially this heading could encompass just about anything that the patient is in contact with that may cause harm or illness. As with RLT's 'maintaining a safe environment', both the internal and the external environments need to be considered; external means the space outside the individual, to include the immediate space and extending to global dimensions, and internal refers to the space inside the individual. The internal environment also includes the psychological and cognitive (thought) processes and factors that influence how people react to hazards, for example their health beliefs, values and knowledge about disease.

Prevention of hazards to human life, human functioning and human well-being is concerned with issues such as hand washing and cross-infection, housing conditions, environmental pollution, poverty and social deprivation, and global influences such as world economy, war and the effects of global warming. Being aware of dangers to the internal environment is concerned with homeostasis within the individual; therefore, maintaining an optimum temperature, hormone and chemical imbalances, bleeding, pain and disruptions to vital signs or any of the systems would be included in this category. Measurements that may be included under this USCR may include estimation of blood glucose, core temperature and localised temperature changes that occur to the skin and tissues indicating infection. Skin that becomes warm to the touch and red or inflamed should be noted, along with any sweating, flushing and shivering.

8. Promotion of human functioning and development within social groups in accordance with human potential, known human limitations and the desire for 'normalcy'

This USCR refers to people's ability to regulate themselves physically, psychologically and socially. It also refers to the individual's drive to maintain and promote their structure and function and their own development.

In other words, this USCR requires you to explore the person's self-concept, how they view themselves and how they interact within society as an autonomous or self-directing being. This would also include role concept: how people see themselves functioning within their family and social group and within society. For example, some people define themselves as 'the bread-winner' in a family and if, through illness or disability, they were no longer able to work, this could have a profound effect on their ability to maintain their own functioning and development. The issues included in RLT's activities of expressing sexuality and dying would be explored under this heading. Information that relates to establishing and maintaining sexual health would include knowledge and understanding of reproduction, contraception and safe sex, puberty, menstruation and menopause. Feeling comfortable with your sexual identity, being able to express your sexuality in the way you dress and your personal appearance, make-up, hairstyle and perfume may be considered, as they all link into a person's self-concept. Information should be gathered that relates to the act of dying – thoughts, fears, concerns, treatments, general beliefs, religious beliefs, spiritual beliefs, rituals, requests and personal wishes.

This USCR is intimately linked with all of the other USCRs. In order for people to maintain and promote their own structure, function and development they need to have the knowledge, skills, motivation and behaviours to attend to the other USCRs. For example, to maintain promotion of normalcy relating to human functioning in excessively hot weather, a person would need to drink more water in order to prevent dehydration. If a person becomes excessively tired, this may lead to psychological stress. If a person is suffering from depression they may become socially isolated. If a hazard is identified, it can then be corrected (if the person has the knowledge, skill, motivation or behaviour to do so) and a balance is maintained.

Now try Activity 4.2.

Activity 4.2

As you can see, there are many similarities between Orem's universal self-care requisites and Roper, Logan and Tierney's activities of living. Can you think why this may be?

How did you do with Activity 4.2? Both models are being used to categorise information about people. There is recognition that, whilst every person is unique, there are enough similarities to be able to put information about all people into either the activities of living or the universal self-care requisites. Using such a framework enables the nurse to develop a holistic and comprehensive assessment. These ideas will be explored further in the critique of the model at the end of the chapter.

Developmental self-care requisites

Each individual develops as a separate, unique person in society.
(Orem, 2001, p. 230)

Orem (2001) recognised that development of a person is concerned with the individual moving through the stages of the lifespan, moving from birth to old age, along with life events such as pregnancy, retirement, loss of people and possessions, health and impending death. The developmental stages have been identified by Orem as:

1. intrauterine life (life in the uterus, prior to birth) and birth;
2. immediately after birth;
3. infancy;
4. childhood, adolescence and entry into adulthood;
5. adulthood;
6. pregnancy.

Looking at theorists such as Erikson (1980) may help us to identify the stages of childhood and adulthood and understand that the experiences at each stage may differ; being an adult of 21 is not the same as being an adult of 90 years of age. The self-care model requires nurses to consider factors that promote positive physical, psychological and social development, as well as factors that may interfere with positive development and how people engage in self-development throughout their lives.

Factors that promote positive physical, psychological and social development

Adults are expected to provide the right environment to promote physical, psychological and social development for themselves and their dependants. When you are a child, you need to receive food with the appropriate amount and balance of nutrients for your physical and mental growth and development. As children are not completely self-caring and therefore unable to do this for themselves, they rely on an adult to provide dependent-care. Children are also reliant upon adults to provide conditions that encourage positive social development. This would involve taking them to playgroups to interact with other children, teaching board games to help them to take turns and to learn how to cooperate with others, and encouraging language development by reading and talking to them. Equally, children are reliant on adults to provide them with a safe environment, or, as Orem suggests, preventing hazards to human life, human functioning and human well-being. This includes protecting them from physical harm, for example putting covers over electric sockets, and also protecting them from emotional harm, by providing a loving and secure relationship.

How people engage in self-development

Orem expected most healthy adults to be able to provide optimum (most favourable) conditions to continue with their own development and maintain their own functioning and well-being. She stated that this demands 'the deliberate involvement of the self in processes of development' (Orem 2001, p. 231).

This includes the development of self-reflection, the development of a positive sense of self-concept, understanding of the role you have to play in society, development of a positive set of values, such as honesty, trust, abiding by laws etc., and development of life goals. The life goals could include becoming a registered nurse, having children or buying a house.

Factors that may interfere with positive development

In order to continue with positive development, you need to recognise and avoid factors that interfere with the process, or overcome or mitigate (lessen) them if they do occur. For example, the loss of a relative or close friend could have an effect on someone's life goals; poor health may have an effect on someone's ability to maintain their physical development; and educational deprivation may have an effect on someone's ability to engage in productive work.

Have a go at Activity 4.3.

Activity 4.3

Think back to when you were growing up and try to identify some of the factors that helped with your physical, psychological and social development. Can you think of any factors that interfered with your positive development? Finally, can you identify two of your current main life goals?

Health deviation self-care requisites (HDSCRs)

Orem argued that, in order for the individual to remain healthy and self-caring, they need to maintain a balance between the demands that are placed upon them and their ability to meet these. When an extra demand is placed upon the person, for example by illness, injury or disease, this is called a health deviation self-care requisite (HDSCR).

Three types of HDSCR are identified by Orem (2001):

+ those relating to changes in a person's physical structure (such as a cut or a broken bone);
+ those relating to changes in physical function (such as inability to maintain blood glucose due to diabetes mellitus);
+ those connected to changes in behaviour and habits of daily living (such as increased alcohol intake or withdrawal from social occasions).

The extra demand placed upon a person by the introduction of a HDSCR may mean that they cannot remain self-caring. It may be possible for individuals to increase their capacity for self-care by calling upon their own reserves. This may be achieved by increasing their knowledge, learning a new skill, changing their behaviour or increasing their motivation. If they are unable to meet the demand then a self-care deficit is said to exist. Sometimes, a relative or friend is able to support them in dependent care by helping them to close the gap between what they are able to do and what they need to do, therefore reducing or removing the deficit. If the deficit cannot be addressed by the patient or significant other, then there is a need for nursing intervention – the nursing agency we discussed earlier in the chapter. Now look at Activity 4.4.

Activity 4.4

Consider the scenario for George Brown in Appendix B. Can you identify the type of health deviation self-care requisites that are causing George's self-care deficits? Try to identify the universal self-care requisites that these HDSCRs are affecting.

How did you do with Activity 4.4? Your examples may have included that George had a HDSCR due to bowel cancer, which required **resection** of the colon. This has led to a change in the

Resection is the surgical removal of some or all of an organ or structure within the body.

structure and the function of the bowel, causing frequent bowel movements for George; this is a self-care deficit in the USCR of satisfactory elimanitive functions. Another HDSCR for George is the presence of cancer, which has spread from the prostate gland. This has caused a change in structure and function of the urinary and reproductive system, leading to George having difficulty passing urine and discomfort due to swelling of the testes and penis. Difficulty in passing urine is also a deficit in the USCR of satisfactory elimanitive functions, but the pain that results from the swelling in the testes and penis causes a deficit in the USCR of prevention of human hazards. Also, as a result of the pain, there has been a change in behaviour: George has changed from being a sociable and communicative person to being withdrawn and 'fed-up', and switching off his hearing aid. These observations and self-statements would be categorised under the USCR of solitude and social interaction. For further examples and information, see the full assessment of George in the scenario using Orem's model in Appendix B.

Helping methods and the nursing systems

When a self-care deficit exists and the individual is no longer able to self-care, then nursing intervention is required. The interventions that can be used by nurses include five different helping methods that can be used to overcome the self-care deficit:

+ acting for or doing for another;
+ guiding and directing;
+ providing physical or psychological support;
+ providing and maintaining an environment that supports personal development;
+ teaching another.

Acting for or doing for another

This helping method should be used only when there is no other alternative to promote self-care. It may be used for babies, children and acutely ill people to address some or all of their universal self-care requisites. For example, a patient returning from a major operation may require a bed bath on the first postoperative day; the nurse would be acting for the patient as they would be unable to self-care at this time.

Guiding and directing

This helping method is used to help people make choices or to help them to do something with which they require supervision. It is often used with the helping method of providing support. This could be used when encouraging someone to change a colostomy bag for the first time; the person has been taught the skill but needs to be supervised as they perform the task.

Providing physical or psychological support

Psychological support may be offered to the patient in a number of ways. Sometimes the mere presence of a nurse is enough to alleviate fear and anxieties. At other times the nurse may need to play a more active role and provide more extensive support, in the form of talking, counselling and therapies. The nurse may also offer physical support at this time by holding something for the patient or giving other practical assistance. Nurses may also offer material resources to a person, such as providing continence appliances and aids.

Providing and maintaining an environment that supports personal development

This requires nurses to provide, or help to provide, the necessary physical and psychological environment to enable people to achieve their goals of care. It may literally be providing a certain type of environment, such as a swimming pool for hydrotherapy, or assisting the individual to change their internal environment by altering a person's attitude towards safe sex.

Teaching another

This method may involve helping a person to gain knowledge or teaching them a skill. It may not be limited to a formal teaching session but can also be carried out in an informal way, when people ask questions or when nurses explain their actions. Teaching people to inject their own insulin would require teaching knowledge and a skill. Often this method is linked with providing an environment that supports personal development.

The five helping methods may all be used during the care of a patient; alternatively just one may be used. Some patients may require different help at different points in their illness. These helping methods are used in conjunction with three nursing systems. The first of these is wholly compensatory, when the nurse compensates completely for the patient's inability to self-care, for example in an intensive care unit. The second nursing system is partially compensatory, when a nurse performs some activities to compensate for limited self-care, for example in a rehabilitation unit. Finally there is supportive-educative, when the patient is self-caring, but requires education or support from the nurse in order to continue to learn and develop new self-care abilities, for example when the nurse gives health promotion advice. Wholly compensatory care may not just be about giving physical care but may also require the nurse to support and protect the patient and/or to make reasoned judgements and decisions for patients who are unable to do so for themselves. A patient may move from needing one system to another, or require more than one system to be used at one time, depending on whether their condition changes.

Think about Practice example 4.2.

Practice example 4.2

When a patient has had a **cerebrovascular accident (CVA)**, they will require wholly compensatory care whilst they are unconscious for many of the USCRs, because they are unable to self-care. As the patient improves and regains consciousness, they may require partially compensatory care, as their movement returns and they are able to perform some of their self-care measures with assistance from the nurse. At the same time the supportive-educative system may be being used, with the nurse offering guidance and support or teaching, or provision of a developmental environment to the patient. In time the patient may move to the educative-supportive system alone.

Cerebrovascular accident (CVA) (sometimes referred to as 'stroke') is a condition of the brain caused by a blood clot or haemorrhage.

Strengths of the model

Orem's Self-Care Model is a fairly widely used model and appears to be applicable to a wide number of practice settings; for example, you may see this model used in a care of the elderly ward, in a surgical ward or in the community.

The model does put the patient at the centre of the process of care planning and this fits well with the views of the NMC (2008) and the Department of Health (2010) requiring nurses to give client-centred care. There's also little doubt that the philosophy of self-care feels 'right' in relation to providing nursing care. When we meet patients for the first time, the instinct is to try and find out what they are able to do for themselves, and structure our care around that.

Orem has contributed to identifying what nurses do uniquely in providing healthcare to patients and has promoted the importance of the patient's own contribution in that care. Whilst the language that she uses can be a little off-putting, she does explain most of the terms that the model is based upon.

Limitations of the model

The model can be a little difficult to understand for UK nurses due to the language used, which contains a lot of 'Americanisms' and is academic in nature. Whilst terms are explained, some remain difficult for UK audiences.

It is not always obvious, especially to the novice nurse, which USCR the information should be categorised under. This requires some experience and discussion about the model for nurses to become confident to use it (Cavanagh 1991). Fawcett (1984) suggests that, although it is claimed to be a holistic model, cultural and socioeconomic aspects are not fully explored by Orem.

The philosophy of self-care may be more suited to the USA rather than Britain, in the emphasis to look after your own health (be self-caring). The USA relies on citizens taking out private health insurance and being responsible for their own healthcare, whereas in Britain there is still a reliance on the National Health Service to look after people from the 'cradle to the grave'.

Conclusion

Orem's Self-Care Model provides an alternative viewpoint on the needs of patients and the role of nurses. Although the focus is on self- and dependent care, the model can be used in any clinical setting for patients with any level of ill-health.

Further reading

As with the other chapters exploring nursing models, our recommendation for those of you who wish to explore models further is to go to the primary source. In this case, that is Orem's own book:

Orem, DE (2001) *Nursing: Concepts of Practice*, 5th ed. St Louis: CV Mosby.

If you want another book that summarises the key elements of a whole range of nursing models – including Orem – then we would recommend that you try:

Aggleton P, Chalmers H (2000) *Nursing Models and Nursing Practice*, 2nd ed. Basingstoke: Macmillan Press.

Chapter 5
The Neuman Systems Model

Why this chapter matters

In the previous two chapters, you've been introduced to two very popular nursing models – Roper, Logan and Tierney's Activities of Living Model and Orem's Self-Care Model. The reason for introducing you to a third example of a nursing model – the Neuman Systems Model – is to give you a wider range of ideas about what nursing actually is and how you can approach care planning and delivery. It all goes back to the point made in Chapter 3: nursing models are tools that you can use, and the more tools you have to choose from, the more likely it is that you will find the best one for the job.

By the end of this chapter, you will be able to:

+ describe the basic features of the Neuman Systems Model;
+ be able to use the Neuman Systems Model to plan care for one of your patients.

Introduction to the model

The Neuman Systems Model was developed in the USA by a nurse academic called Betty Neuman. Neuman wanted to develop an educational framework that would help her nursing students better understand issues surrounding health and care. This led her to first develop a model in 1970 (Neuman, 2010b). Neuman's broad philosophy is similar to that of the Roper, Logan and Tierney model discussed in Chapter 3, in the sense that she wanted to move away from a traditional 'illness' model to one that considers the 'total person'. However, what Neuman did rather more comprehensively than Roper, Logan and Tierney was to expand the use of the model to embrace families, groups and the wider community. Neuman refers to her model as the 'systems model': it offers an interdisciplinary approach that is not restricted just to nurses. The model stresses the complementary work of healthcare professionals and can be used by anyone working in the healthcare setting. Despite the model first being developed decades ago, it has continued to evolve and the ideas are very much in keeping with today's health and social care policies that encourage multidisciplinary care, health education and promotion of 'wellness'.

The model is based on three particular theories – stress adaptation theory, gestalt theory and systems theory. A brief outline of each of these may help you to understand the fundamental principles that drive the use of the model.

Stress adaptation theory

At one time or another, we will tell our friends and families that we are under a lot of stress. As a society, we are told by the media that more and more of us suffer the effects of stress. But what exactly do we mean by 'stress'? To many people, the term could relate to things like a gas bill, an exam or a job interview. Each of these might be referred to as a **stimulus**. Some of us would argue that stress is a feeling or set of behaviours including panic, sweaty palms, or an increase in breathing and heart rate. Feelings or behaviours like this are sometimes known as **responses**. The idea of stimuli causing responses formed the basis of theories of stress for many years, but it does have limitations. The problem is that not everyone feels stressed at the thought of an unpaid bill, an exam or a job interview. You may have friends with seemingly insurmountable problems who appear very relaxed and 'stress-free'. Equally, you may know people who don't appear to have many problems, but who tell you that they cannot cope and show all the signs of a stress response.

To deal with some of these issues, Cox (1978) offers the transactional model. This model suggests that stress is an imbalance between demands made on the individual and their perceived ability to cope or adapt to it. Put simply, when you are faced with a **stressor**, you evaluate it and then assess your own available coping strategies and resources. A state of stress occurs only when you perceive the threat to be greater than the resources that are available to you. To use the example of the exam, if you are confident that you have the knowledge to pass easily, you are unlikely to be stressed. If you don't think that you have the ability to answer the questions, you will feel under stress.

Whether other people judge your assessment to be accurate or not is irrelevant; it is your perception that decides whether the stress response is triggered or not. Stressors cannot be specified by their physical characteristics, only by their consequences as perceived by you or any other individual. Spiders are a simple example of this: show two people the same spider (that is, the same stressor), and you may get two different responses – one person may smile happily at it, and the other may run away screaming. Equally, each patient you care for is unique and has their own reactions to stressors, governed by their interpretation of the stressor and their ability to cope. So, for example, you may have two patients awaiting the same

A **stimulus** is something that provokes a reaction.

A **response** is an observable reaction to a stimulus.

A **stressor** is something that may cause stress.

surgical procedure, but one will be very calm and relaxed whilst the other may be petrified – this is why an individualised assessment is such an important element of your care. This is a brief outline of the theory that underpins the stress adaptation theory but, if you want to read more about the theories of stress, then Wilson (2005) offers a more detailed account.

Gestalt theory

The gestalt psychologists were some of the earliest theorists to consider how our brains process information and make sense of it. They concentrated on explanations that argued that 'the whole is greater than the sum of the parts'. This statement means that it doesn't matter what you are looking at; you cannot make sense of it if you are looking at the individual parts as separate components, because the whole picture is always more complex than the individual parts put together. Think about your favourite band and compare one of their songs to a piece of classical music. Both pieces of music played as a 'whole' will obviously sound completely different, and will probably have a different effect on you. You certainly wouldn't have any difficulty in telling the two apart. However, if you were to break down the two pieces of music into their constituent parts – that is, collate all the individual notes (Bs, Cs, Ds etc.) into groups – do you think that you could differentiate between the two so easily? It is when the notes are put together in a particular way that the two pieces of music become so different: the whole is greater than the sum of its parts. A melody is more than a set of individual notes; it is the relationship of the notes together that creates the tune, just as a book is more than letters, words and sentences.

Similarly, when we consider individuals, there is perhaps little difference between two people in terms of their constituent atoms, cells, chemicals and physiological structure but enormous differences between the two individuals when all the parts are put together to make a whole person.

Systems theory

If your best friend was in a particularly bad mood this morning, what reasons might you look for to explain this? It could be because of some sort of internal physical disturbance or imbalance. For example, her blood sugar might be low because she didn't get the chance to eat breakfast, or she might be at the stage of her menstrual cycle when she often feels a bit sensitive. She might even have a hangover from the night before. Equally, her mood could reflect some events that affected her this morning, such as an argument with her partner, trouble getting her children ready in time for school, or the washing machine flooding the floor. Maybe she went to her car this morning and found that she had a flat tyre, which resulted in her being late for work. She may have arrived at work to find an email banning overtime and proposing redundancies because of spending cuts. This might particularly worry her because the latest rumour in the business pages of her newspaper is that energy costs are set to rise in response to global financial turmoil, putting even more pressure on her family's finances. In fact, all these things might have happened, in which case you can probably forgive her for being a bit tetchy.

Systems analysis argues that, in order to understand your friend's behaviour, you have to look beyond just the individual and her immediate environment. You have to look beyond the interactions that she has with her family and neighbourhood, and towards the larger frameworks within which she finds herself (e.g. her place of work, country of residence and global influences). A comprehensive understanding cannot come from looking at the separate components: remember, the gestalt theory suggests that the whole is greater than the sum of the parts.

Systems theory argues that all of nature is arranged at different levels and is made up of smaller systems within larger systems. We can see this when we consider the scenario above, with each level reflecting distinctive properties and characteristics. Your friend is a complex system, made up of lots of little systems. She also exists in different systems, such as her family, her home town, her workplace and the global system. Each system is an entity in itself but also makes up a part of a larger system. Nothing exists in isolation and everything is interrelated and interdependent. In other words, if you want to look at why your friend is snappy, you could look for an answer based on each of the levels in isolation, from her internal environment (blood sugar and hormones) right up to the global level (worrying about the state of the economy.) However, influences within each level contribute to her mood, and it would be meaningless to consider the levels individually and in isolation. It is when you put all the components together that you get a full picture of why she is behaving as she is, and why she needs your support.

The idea that everything is interrelated and interdependent means that a change or disturbance in any one system will have an effect on all other parts of that system and may subsequently affect other systems. It is like throwing a stone in a pool of still water: the ripples start at the centre and spread outwards in ever increasing circles. The effect of one part of the system will reverberate and affect all the other parts, spreading outwards and inwards.

Before moving on, let's think of a healthcare example to demonstrate systems theory. One of the most obvious systems within healthcare is a hospital, and a change in one part of this system will often affect many other parts. For example, imagine that a nurse within an intensive care unit (ICU) is off sick at short notice. Because this nurse is off sick, an ICU bed has to stay closed as there is no one to staff it. Because this bed is closed, a patient due to go for surgery today has to have their operation cancelled because they have no ICU bed to go to afterwards. Because the patient's surgery is cancelled, they will not be leaving the ward today, so their bed won't be freed up. This means that the patient due to go to that bed from the Accident and Emergency (A&E) department can't be transferred into it, meaning that they will have to stay in the department for longer than planned. This is just one simple example of how altering one part of a system – an ICU nurse being off sick – can cause a problem in an entirely different part of the system – a patient staying longer than planned in A&E.

WHAT HAVE YOU LEARNT SO FAR?

+ The Neuman Systems Model was first developed in 1970 in the USA.
+ The model links into stress adaptation theory, which explores how we respond to different stimuli.
+ The model also relates to gestalt theory, which suggests that the sum is greater than the constituent parts.
+ Systems theory, which underpins Neuman's ideas, suggests that we are all interrelated systems, operating at many different levels. A change in one part of a system is likely to cause disruption to many different parts of the system.

Key elements of the model

There's much more to Neuman's model than just those three ideas summarised above, but you'll see the key ideas from stress adaptation theories, gestalt theory and systems theory popping up at regular intervals as we look at the model in more detail. First of all, we'll consider what the model has to say about the person, the environment and health.

The person

Neuman refers to individuals requiring help with their health as clients rather than patients. People are seen as 'open systems' that are in constant interaction with their environment, making all of us susceptible to all manner of stressors. The focus for using Neuman's model is on establishing how we react and adapt to any disruption of the system caused by stressors and how we try and maintain a balance (or equilibrium) between the environment and ourselves. It's important to realise that disruption of our system is not always a bad thing, because it can act as a driving force to motivate us, sometimes forcing us to change and develop for the better. For example, being made redundant will cause a huge disruption, but for some people (though by no means all) it provides an impetus for them to make a positive change in their life, such as embarking on a new career.

Variable areas

According to Neuman, each of us has five 'variable areas', which interact with each other. These are:

+ **Physiological:** these might include our anatomical structures, physiological processes and genetic factors
+ **Psychological:** including mental processes such as language, memory, intelligence, temperament, personality and body image
+ **Sociocultural**: areas that can relate to things such as social class, ethnic origin, beliefs, values and norms
+ **Developmental:** the physical and psychosocial changes that occur as we pass through the different developmental stages, such as puberty and the menopause
+ **Spiritual:** relating to our spiritual and religious beliefs

The model represents the client as a series of concentric circles surrounding a basic core structure, giving us something like a two-dimensional Russian doll, where the different smaller sized dolls are all stacked inside of each other to make up the one larger doll (see Figure 5.1).

The basic structure

The 'basic structure' represents a person's energy source and is the very essence of who and what we all are. It is made up of common features or survival factors which fall under the same sub-headings of the five variable areas discussed above.

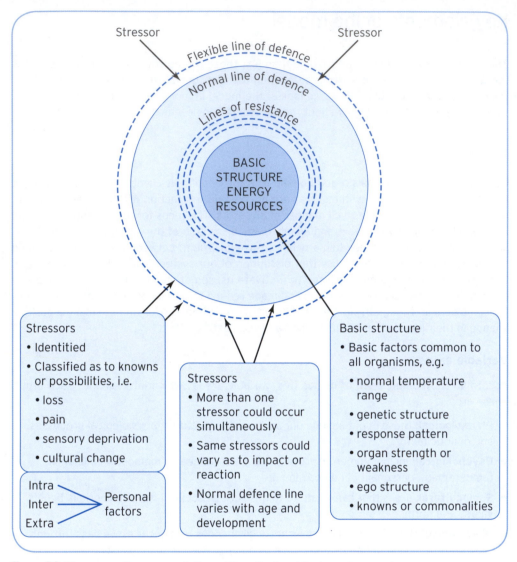

Figure 5.1 Diagrammatic representation of the client and their environment.
From Neuman B (2002) The Neuman Systems Model. In Neuman B, Fawcett J (2002)
The Neuman Systems Model, 4th ed. New Jersey: Prentice Hall.

Some of the features within the basic structure are shared by all people – for example, we all have a circulatory system, and we all use language. However, within these common features, there are individual variations. For example, in relation to the circulatory system, we might be predisposed to having **hypertension**. In terms of language, people will speak in different languages, with different regional dialects, different accents and different pace and volume. Some of these differences within common features will be due to genetic factors, whilst others are as a result of our upbringing.

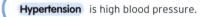 **Hypertension** is high blood pressure.

Lines of resistance

Outside the basic structure are three boundaries, starting with the lines of resistance. These lines surround the basic structure in order to protect it from the attack by stressors and to help us maintain internal harmony and stability. The lines of resistance are essentially the resources that we have available to deal with attacks by stressors, and are linked to the five variable areas listed earlier (physiological, psychological, sociocultural, developmental and spiritual). Some of the lines of resistance are 'built in' from the time that we are born – for example, the ability of our blood to clot when we cut ourselves. Other elements of the lines of resistance may be acquired as a result of the responses and changes (adaptations) that we make as a result of previous experiences. One example might be the response of our immune system to an infection that we have either had before or have been immunised against. If the lines of resistance are effective (e.g. if our blood clots or if our immune system fights off the infection), then the system will 'deflect' the stressor. If the lines of resistance fail, they will allow the stressor to breach the core structure and will lead to a depletion of our energy. If energy continues to be depleted, then this can cause death. Consider Activity 5.1.

Activity 5.1

Think about you and your life. List the lines of resistance that you think you were born with and those that you have acquired as a result of your experiences and circumstances. Remember, they are related to the five variable areas so use them as a guide to help you identify them.

How did you do with Activity 5.1? Did your examples include any of the following?

+ **Physiological:** one of the best examples of a physiological line of resistance that we've already mentioned is related to immunity to disease that you might have developed through previous exposure or planned immunisation. You may also have built up physiological lines of resistance by eating a healthy diet or keeping yourself physically fit.
+ **Psychological:** throughout your life, you will have built up a number of psychological lines of resistance. These might include your level of intelligence, learnt behaviours, coping strategies (such as exam technique or ways of enhancing your body image) or your personality.
+ **Sociocultural:** your sociocultural status may provide you with lines of resistance against stressors. You may have a close circle of friends and an active social life. You may have a number of hobbies and interests, a long-term relationship or even a lot of disposable income. All these things help you deal with day-to-day stressors.
+ **Developmental:** our lines of resistance often become stronger as we move through the different developmental stages. For example, we all become more physically developed as we move towards adulthood, and we also gain sexual and emotional maturity. Conversely, as we continue to move through developmental stages, our lines of resistance may become weaker due to the ageing process.
+ **Spiritual:** many of us develop lines of resistance through spiritual and religious means. Examples might include membership of a formalised religion, or spiritual support through groups, reading or study.

Normal line of defence

The normal line of defence is created from the lines of resistance and is drawn as a solid circle surrounding them (see Figure 5.1). It represents a person's health status that has developed over time. Put more simply, it reflects how well someone usually is and gives us all a baseline to compare our current state of health against. Although your level of wellness is relatively stable, it does have the ability to change over time. For example, if you don't normally have back pain, then the presence of such a stressor will be seen – quite rightly – as an aberration from the norm that needs addressing. However, if you have had years of chronic back pain, then your normal line of defence changes to reflect this – the presence of back pain becomes 'normal' to you. Our normal line of resistance also changes as we get older, with our 'baseline' state of health and fitness generally becoming less good due to the ageing process.

Flexible line of defence

The flexible line of defence is represented as a broken line surrounding the normal line of defence and forms the first line of protection against attack from the different stressors. It is sometimes described as a 'buffer' that protects the normal line of defence. It is seen as temporary in nature and as such is not as stable as the lines of resistance. Neuman (2010b) describes it as being similar to an accordion because it can move in and out, varying from day to day, affected by factors such as how tired we are, how well we are eating and what our psychological mood is. Once the line of defence is penetrated, the individual presents with symptoms of instability or illness. There are an enormous number of things that can affect the flexible line of defence, but here are a few examples:

+ **Physiological:** the strength and state of the immune system can be affected by lack of sleep, poor diet or extreme cold or heat. Our energy levels can be affected by low blood sugar levels, our level of hydration is affected by not drinking enough, and fitness levels can be lowered by minor injury or overuse of muscles.

+ **Psychological:** a person's body image – often something that strengthens our structure – can be affected by surgery, an inability to meet hygiene needs, or illness. Our emotional stability can be affected by alcohol and other drugs, relationship problems or lack of sleep.

+ **Sociocultural:** our ability to cope with stressors might be enhanced by getting a pay rise or winning some money on the lottery. Equally, we might be less able to cope if we have recently had to give up a recreational activity or suffered bereavement.

+ **Developmental:** our flexible line of defence will be affected by developmental issues such as puberty, pregnancy, the menopause and old age.

+ **Spiritual:** the strengthening or weakening of one's faith may have an impact on the flexible line of defence – that is, the ability to cope with stressors.

Have a go at Activity 5.2.

Activity 5.2

Consider the scenario of Shoaib Hameed in Appendix C. Can you identify the factors that are influencing Shoaib's flexible line of defence?

How did you do with Activity 5.2? There are a number of things that might have affected Shoaib's flexible line of defence. For example, the fact that he works long hours, has a rather poor relationship with his family and has an 'unhealthy' lifestyle have made him more susceptible to cardiovascular disease. In addition, the myocardial infarction that he has suffered has now further affected his ability to deal with stressors, and has therefore (in Neuman speak) moved the flexible line of defence closer to the normal line of defence.

The environment

Neuman suggests that we have three environments to consider when planning and providing healthcare.

+ **Internal environment:** this represents all the influences that are within us (e.g. our genetic information, anatomical and physiological features).

+ **External environment:** as the name suggests, these are all the influences outside us (e.g. other people, our workplace, the global economy).

+ **Created environment:** Neuman describes the created environment as a 'symbolic expression of system wholeness'. Slightly more helpfully, she goes on to describe the created environment as something related to coping strategies. The simplest way of thinking of the created environment is as mechanisms that we develop and unconsciously use to cope with stressors (e.g. putting on extra clothes when we have a cold, or maintaining a positive outlook on life).

Stressors and responses

The Neuman Systems Model suggests that all of us are constantly confronted with environmental stressors that can produce disruption to our system (Skalski et al. 2006). Stressors come in many different shapes and sizes, and will have an individual meaning for different people. This links back to the idea that we discussed earlier in relation to stress adaptation theory, where we highlighted that a person's response to a stressor is much more important than the stressor itself. This means that, as a nurse, it is important to try to view any situation from the patient's viewpoint as well as your own. One important thing to note is that stressors don't always have a negative effect: some actually bring about positive change and act as a motivational force, energising the individual. However, where stressors may impart a negative effect on the patient, it is the lines of defence that respond to the stressors to prevent them from reaching the basic structure.

Stressors can be divided into three categories.

+ **Intrapersonal stressors:** these involve the internal environment and refer to stressors that occur within the individual, such as disease, infection, trauma, grief, anxiety, loss, pain, role change, developmental changes, puberty, menopause and a crisis of faith.

+ **Interpersonal stressors:** these involve the immediate environment and refer to stressors that occur between one or more individuals, such as conflict or change between family members, neighbours or friends, marriage, parenthood, divorce, role change, role conflict, racism, ageism and sexism.

+ **Extrapersonal stressors:** these involve the external environment and structures that impact on the individual; the stressors occur outside of individual and immediate relationships. Extrapersonal stressors can include poverty, deprivation, pollution, climate change, unemployment due to recession, political changes and policies affecting health resources and lack of education.

The response of a person to a stressor varies from individual to individual and very much depends on the level of disruption occurring within the system and how effective the lines of defence are in that particular situation. Again, the responses relate to the five variable areas and can occur at intra-, inter- and extrapersonal level:

+ **Intrapersonal responses:** these might include pathological responses such as inflammation, clotting of blood or shock. Stressors may also cause intrapersonal responses such as anxiety, lack of sleep, depression, aggression, violence, comfort eating or spending of money ('retail therapy').

+ **Interpersonal responses:** stressors may cause a number of interpersonal responses such as arguments or even violence between family and friends. Over time, stressors may cause permanent breakdowns in relationships.

+ **Extrapersonal responses:** some stressors may cause extrapersonal responses such as campaigning for or against a certain cause, creative activities, turning away from religion and belief systems, or even committing a criminal offence.

Now think about Activity 5.3.

Activity 5.3

Have another look at the scenario for Suzy Clarke in Appendix A. What sorts of stressors (intrapersonal, interpersonal or extrapersonal) are affecting Suzy, and how has she responded?

If you've had a go at Activity 5.3, you will have seen that Suzy has certainly been affected by a range of different stressors, including lack of money (extrapersonal) and problems with her friends (interpersonal). She has also demonstrated many different responses, including eating a poor diet, smoking and suffering panic attacks – which are all intrapersonal. She has also shown some extrapersonal responses – problems completing her university work, threatening her continuation on the programme.

One of the interesting elements of thinking about people in terms of stressors and responses is that, often, a response can itself become a stressor. In Suzy's case, the combination of her friends, her university work and her lack of money (the stressors) caused the panic attacks (a response). Because she is worried about the health implications of the panic attacks, they have in themselves become a stressor that needs addressing.

Health

Neuman views health as a continuum: as we move away from being as healthy as we can be – 'optimal wellness' – we get sicker and sicker until we reach the other end of the continuum and die.

Neuman's ideas about levels of wellness are linked to energy levels: a person's point on the continuum relates to the amount of available energy in their system. If our body system is able to produce more energy than it expends, then we feel well. If we expend more energy than we are able to produce, then we become unwell and, if the net loss of energy continues unabated, we die. These changes in energy flow are usually caused by the impact of stressors – for example, exposure to a virus causes our bodies to use more energy to try to fight the infection. This energy is required to try to return the system to a state of stability. Once we've fought off the infection (i.e. restored stability), energy usage will fall below energy generation, and we gradually feel better – so 'wellness' is a reflection of the system's stability and reaction to stressors.

Goals of nursing

The main goal of nursing is to help the patient reach their full health potential by delivering interventions that strengthen the patient's responses, or decrease the impact of the stressors.

Neuman discusses three types of nursing intervention that can be utilised to help patients achieve their optimal state of wellness. These fall under the broad heading of 'prevention-as-intervention', and are specifically primary, secondary and tertiary prevention. We'll talk about these in much more detail in Chapter 11, but it is worth summarising exactly what Neuman means by each.

Primary prevention

This type of intervention occurs when a stressor is suspected or identified before a reaction has occurred within the system. The goal is to reduce the possibility of contact with a stressor and to strengthen the line of defence. A good example of primary prevention as intervention is health promotion. If you have a patient whom you recognise is at risk of heart disease (the stressor), then you try to help the patient change their lifestyle to reduce the chance of problems developing in the future.

Secondary prevention

This type of intervention occurs after a stressor has crossed the line of defence and has caused a reaction. The goal of secondary prevention as intervention is to help the patient to stabilise and return to their 'normal' state of health. To do this, you will treat the patient's symptoms and support them while they get better.

Tertiary prevention

Tertiary prevention as intervention occurs after the treatment stage and involves helping the client to maintain or stabilise their health state to avoid a possible recurrence of the crisis. In simple terms, these interventions can be thought of as rehabilitation and preventing the problems happening again.

Strengths of the model

The ideas within the Neuman Systems Model have produced a wealth of nursing research and have been used widely in nurse education. Clinically, the model is one of the most popular and commonly used in the USA (August-Brady 2000). Even though the Neuman Systems

Model is by no means the most widely used in the UK, it does have a number of characteristics that are relevant to healthcare today. For example, emphasis is clearly placed on primary prevention as a possible intervention, a directive that is echoed in policy directed towards targets linked to reducing smoking and obesity rates. Tertiary prevention deals with helping patients to return to their normal state of well-being after treatment or to cope with continuing care needs that result from the illness. This also has parallels with the increasing focus on reablement and long-term disease management.

One of the broad ideas underpinning the model – the fact that we have defences against stressors that enable us to protect ourselves against illness – is easily applicable to many areas of nursing practice and research, and this contributes further to the popularity of Neuman's framework. For example, a recent piece of nursing research surrounding vitamin D deficiency in people with **glioma** used Neuman's model to conceptualise vitamin D as one of the lines of resistance that can help the body recover from cancer (Rice *et al.*, 2010).

The assessment process using Neuman's model – which we deal with in greater detail in Chapter 8 – is less restrictive than some models. It allows the nurse to use clinical judgement to structure the assessment, and places great emphasis on the perceptions of patients themselves.

Finally, some of the principles of the model also seem to intuitively 'fit' with what we know about ourselves and others. For example, some days we are more able to cope with the stresses of life than others – in 'Neuman-speak' our flexible line of defence is sometimes further away from the normal line of defence than others.

Limitations of the model

The model, like many other nursing theories, includes a lot of rather flowery language, making some elements difficult to understand. There is a lack of clarity in some key issues such as the actual meaning of 'created environment' and the difference between 'interpersonal' and 'extrapersonal' stressors.

The detail of the model also contains some unusual elements. For example, when assessing the client, it is stated that only three areas of concern should be identified, but no rationale is given for this. Again, we'll expand on this in Chapter 8.

The variable of spirituality is not, in itself, unusual within a nursing model (RLT and Orem also include reference to spiritual needs), but Neuman does seem to have an explicitly religious agenda. The discussion of the spiritual variable includes terminology such as 'The human spirit combines with the power of the Holy Spirit as a gift from God' (Neuman and Fawcett 2002, p.16). It is unclear how the model can therefore be used to care for patients with different (or no) religious beliefs.

Whilst Neuman suggests that the unique role of the nurse is to care, coordinate and collaborate, some argue that the role is left unclear and fragmented; this means that there is a danger that the model does not define nursing clearly enough.

Glioma is a type of tumour, most commonly found in the brain or spinal column.

Finally, the unstructured nature of assessment may make the model more difficult to use for inexperienced staff. Compared with a rather prescriptive model (e.g. Roper, Logan and Tierney and their activities of living), the systems model does require the nurse to use their clinical judgement more creatively to identify needs.

Conclusion

In the last three chapters, we've introduced you to well-known nursing models. They all have strengths and weaknesses, and you may already have some ideas about which you prefer. The second half of this book applies the three nursing models to care planning, which will enable you to see how some of the concepts we've discussed can be used in practice. You may want to skip straight on to those chapters, but there are a couple more chapters within this section that help 'set the scene' for care planning. Next, we look at different tools that you can use to help you assess your patients.

Further reading

If you want to find out about a model in depth, then the recommended text has to be that written by the 'inventor' of the model. In the case of the systems model, the latest edition of the primary source is;

Neuman B, Fawcett, J (2010) *The Neuman Systems Model*, 5th ed. New Jersey, Prentice Hall.

Not only does this book contain all the details of the model, but it also has an autobiography of Betty Neuman, and a history of the model's development. In addition, there are many chapters by other authors, exploring how the model has been used in practice. Be warned, though: as with many textbooks about nursing models, it can get a bit heavy-going at times!

For those seeking a more interactive experience, there is also a website dedicated to the promotion and advancement of the model: www.neumansystemsmodel.org.

Chapter 6
Assessment tools

Why this chapter matters

During a shift at work, you meet Dean, a 24-year-old man who seems rather unhappy and withdrawn. When you carry out your nursing assessment, you find out that he lost his job six months ago, and now he spends most of his time sitting around the house drinking cider.

After talking to Dean for some time, you suspect that he may be depressed and that he is becoming dependent on alcohol. How could you gather evidence to find out whether this really is the case or not?

This chapter is about assessment tools that would be of use to you in an example such as this. In Dean's case, it might be useful if he was to complete the Hospital Anxiety and Depression Scale (HADS) and the Alcohol Use Disorders Identification Test (AUDIT). Tools are also available that assess physical risk, psychological well-being and social status. Although they are not a replacement for your assessment skills, they are a really useful way of adding to what you know about patients.

By the end of the chapter you will be able to:

+ identify assessment tools that are of particular use to your clinical area;

+ explain to your colleagues the concepts of reliability, validity, sensitivity and specificity;

+ understand the advantages and disadvantages of using assessment tools in nursing.

What are assessment tools?

The types of tool that we're going to talk about in this chapter can be given all sorts of different names. Depending on exactly what they're aimed at doing, the tools can be called assessment scales, risk assessment tools or screening tools. For ease, we'll just call them all 'assessment tools' for the rest of the chapter.

The purpose of assessment tools is to help you do your job more effectively. Chapter 2 has shown how important assessment is as part of planning care – if you don't assess patients properly, then you won't have the information required to identify problems and plan nursing interventions. A lot of your assessment might be based upon your own skills and the model of nursing that you use – we'll talk a lot more about this in Chapter 8. Assessment tools provide a way of gaining additional information that may help you ask the right questions and decide what the answers mean.

The best way of really getting an idea of what we mean by assessment tools is to look at some examples. The tools that we're going to look at are just the tip of the iceberg, but they'll give you some idea of the types of thing that you'll see in practice. Depending on what they are used for, assessment tools can be broadly split into three main types – health screening and diagnosis, description and prediction (Gibbons 1998).

Screening and diagnosis tools try to identify the presence or severity of a particular problem. For example, the Hospital Anxiety and Depression Scale (HADS) has 14 questions that are used to detect whether a patient is suffering from anxiety or depression. It is used throughout healthcare – not just in hospitals, but also as a tool in areas such as general practice (Bjelland et al. 2002). There are other examples of screening tools used in practice. For example, the Alcohol Use Disorders Identification Test (AUDIT) allows healthcare workers to detect the possibility of alcohol problems with 10 simple questions (Reinert and Allen 2007).

In truth, all assessment tools are a bit descriptive, because they allow you to describe the patient's condition to someone else. However, some tools are referred to as purely descriptive because they don't do anything else. Probably the best example of this is the Barthel Activity of Daily Living Index (Mahoney and Barthel 1965). This index gives carers the opportunity to assess a number of different elements of a patient's physical ability. Overall, the score allows you to describe how dependent a patient is – the higher the score someone gets, the less dependent they are (Hartigan and O'Mahony 2011). For this reason, it is often used when deciding on the level of care that someone may need within the community. Just one important point to clarify about the Barthel Index: the Activities of Daily Living (ADLs) described are not the same as the Activities of Living (ALs) described by Roper, Logan and Tierney's model!

One extremely common type of descriptive assessment tool is the Visual Analogue Scale (VAS). A VAS is a line with two extremes of a particular sensation or experience marked. For example, in a pain VAS, one end of the line might refer to 'no pain' whereas the other end of the line will represent 'the worst pain that you can imagine'. The patient makes a mark on the line to represent the level of pain they are feeling. In some scales, the line is marked with numbers so that the patient can give their pain a 'score' between 0 (no pain) and 10 (the worst pain you can imagine). The VAS can also be used for a range of other subjective measurements, including breathlessness, fatigue, nausea and quality of life (Waltz et al. 2010). These types of scales don't really diagnose or predict any elements of the patient's well-being but simply give you an idea of how bad a particular symptom is or how a patient is feeling.

The final type of assessment tool is one that has predictive qualities – that is, it helps you to decide whether someone is likely to develop a problem in the future. There are a whole host of predictive assessment tools that you might use in your practice, but we'll just look at a few. If you work in a hospital, then one of the most common areas in which predictive tools are used is in relation to the prevention of pressure ulcers. A number of different tools exist – the most well-known ones are the Waterlow, Norton and Braden scales – each of which assesses a range of patient characteristics (e.g. age, mobility) to identify the risk of pressure ulcers developing (Anthony et al. 2008).

Assessment tools are available to predict a whole range of other possible problems. For example, the risk of patients falling can be assessed using the STRATIFY tool (Oliver *et al.* 2008). A constipation risk assessment scale (CRAS) has recently been developed (Richmond and Wright 2006), Many hospitals use an 'early warning score' to predict which patients are likely to become critically ill, and there are over 70 tools designed to assess the risk of nutritional problems in patients (Green and Watson 2006). These examples are closely related to the nursing needs of patients, but there are also tools that assess more medical or surgical issues. For example, there are tools that calculate an older person's risk of developing cardiovascular disease (heart disease or stroke) by putting together information about age, gender, smoking habits and blood pressure (Weatherley and Jackson 2011). For patients undergoing cardiac surgery, assessment tools can be used to predict the chances of dying – the mortality risk – during or soon after the operation. To see how this works, go to www.euroscore.org and put in different information to see how the mortality rate alters.

STOP AND THINK

Think about your own workplace. What assessment tools do you use yourself or do you see being used by your colleagues? Are these assessment tools used for screening and diagnosis, description or prediction?

WHAT HAVE YOU LEARNT SO FAR?

+ Assessment tools help you gather information from the patient.
+ Screening tools try to identify the presence of a problem.
+ Descriptive tools help you describe the patient's capabilities or condition to someone else, often in terms of numbers.
+ Predictive tools help you decide whether someone is likely to develop a problem.

We've had a very quick look at the different types of assessment tools that are available, and you've thought of a few that you use at work. The next question that we need to ask ourselves is quite simple – what are the benefits of using assessment tools?

Why are assessment tools so useful?

Assessment tools are used by all healthcare practitioners. Some of the tools that we mentioned above are usually completed only by doctors, some are used by registered nurses, and some can be of use to anybody who looks after patients. Whatever your professional role and specialty, you'll see and use assessment tools regularly, so why are they so popular?

The first reason (and these are in no particular order) is that assessment tools can be very useful to less experienced practitioners. To explore this in a little more detail, we need to look briefly at how nurses make clinical judgements. One of the most famous pieces of nursing research was carried out by an American nurse called Patricia Benner. Benner (1984) produced a piece of work called *From Novice to Expert*, which explored how nurses develop their expertise and decision-making skills. Benner found that nurses very early in their careers – 'novices' – often base their decisions on advice from more experienced nurses. In Benner's work, this is related to asking for advice, but the basic idea fits in very neatly with assessment tools. In developing assessment tools, experienced nurses (and other practitioners) have essentially done your work for you – they have identified key questions that should be asked about a patient, and then provided a judgement about what particular answers mean. From this point of view, assessment tools can be seen as a checklist that must be followed during particular elements of an assessment. Practice example 6.1 demonstrates how an assessment tool can aid a less experienced practitioner.

Practice example 6.1

Dora is a newly qualified nurse working on a rehabilitation ward. The nurse in charge asks Dora to go and assess Mr Claypole, a long-term patient recovering from a stroke. The ward manager thinks that Mr Claypole may be at risk of becoming malnourished and wants Dora to explore his nutritional status.

Being new to the job, Dora is unsure of what questions to ask and how to interpret any findings. Fortunately, the ward uses a nutrition assessment scale to help make decisions about each patient's nutritional status. Dora uses the questions on this scale to get an objective measure of Mr Claypole's risk and finds that he is, indeed, at increased nutritional risk.

Once you become more experienced, you develop more sophisticated clinical decision-making skills and become more expert at identifying problems without needing to follow a very structured checklist of questions. So, if you are an 'expert' practitioner, what extra benefits do assessment tools provide for you?

Well, another reason why assessment tools are so popular in practice is that most of them result in you getting some sort of definite 'score' for the patient. Depending on the type of assessment tool that you use, you might end up with a number that can be related to a level of risk (for example, high, medium or low risk of developing a pressure sore), or a very specific measurement of risk, such as an estimated chance of dying while having an operation. Numbers can be very useful in healthcare. In terms of assessment tools, they can tell you whether someone is improving or not; for example, if my Waterlow scale score was 18 last week and is 14 this week, then it could be argued that at least one aspect of my health is getting better (this links closely to the idea of 'ongoing evaluation' that we discuss in Chapters 2 and 12). Having objective numbers within our assessment can make it easier to identify baselines and set measurable goals for our patients. Numbers also allow you to make decisions about how equipment or services can be shared out amongst patients in the fairest way. Whether we like it or not, there are not always enough resources to go around in healthcare and assessment tools can help you make difficult decisions. Practice example 6.2 carries on the pressure sore theme to show how assessment tools might be used in this way.

So assessment tools can help you to ask the right questions, make decisions about patient risk and target resources effectively. That's all well and good, but we haven't really mentioned the patient yet – how can assessment tools directly help them?

First of all, assessment tools may be useful educational tools for patients. Let's think about those tools that help to predict someone's risk of developing a disease later in life. The example discussed earlier on in the chapter was a set of tables that allow nurses or doctors to give a patient a rough idea of how likely it is that they will develop cardiovascular disease in the next 10 years. Let's imagine that you have a patient in front of you who has a risk of developing cardiovascular disease that is greater than 20 per cent (one in five) in the next 10 years. The assessment tool allows you to show the patient exactly why they are at such high risk. It might be because they smoke, have abnormal levels of cholesterol in their blood, or are overweight. Most importantly, the tools let you show the patient how changing their lifestyle by giving up smoking, losing weight and reducing cholesterol levels will lessen their risk.

Practice example 6.2

Ward 12 is a 24-bedded unit for patients with a range of medical conditions. It has access to six pressure-relieving mattresses, specially designed to reduce the risk of patients developing pressure sores. Each patient who is admitted to the ward has their pressure sore risk assessed using the Waterlow scale.

On a daily basis, the Waterlow scores of patients on the ward are reviewed. Decisions about who should be placed on a pressure-relieving mattress are made on the basis of those who are at greatest risk (that is, those with the highest Waterlow scores). In doing so, the assessment tool allows a limited resource to be given to those patients that need it the most.

Finally, some assessment tools – notably those related to calculating the risk of surgery – will help patients and their families make important decisions about their treatment. Assessment tools may allow doctors to provide patients with estimates of survival rates from certain operations. The patient is then given the information they need to make some stark choices – for example, do they want to continue with chronic pain in their hip, or do they want an operation which carries a one-in-a-hundred chance of dying? These may not be pleasant things to think about, but at least they make sure that patients are given the right information about their options and can therefore give informed consent.

We've discussed how assessment tools provide a whole range of advantages to you, your colleagues and your patients. They help you learn how to assess effectively, let you identify patients at risk, act as an educational tool, and provide people with important information about any procedures that they may need to undergo. But . . . where do they come from, and how do you know that they are accurate? Before we discuss that, spend some time doing a bit of research in your own workplace and try Activity 6.1.

How are assessment tools developed?

If you've completed Activity 6.1, you'll have found out that developing an assessment tool is not simply a case of having a good idea, writing down a few questions, and putting it into practice. Any assessment tool used in practice should be tested in a number of ways to make sure that it does what it is supposed to do. These tests will be designed to evaluate a number of different characteristics, and it is worth looking at each of these in turn. Some of the terms used often crop up in relation to the design of research studies, so you may have heard of them before.

The first thing to think about is reliability. We often use the term reliability in everyday language. Whenever people buy a car, they have a number of reasons for picking a particular model. The last time you bought a car, you may have chosen a particular model because you were told by the salesperson (so it must be true!) that it was very reliable. What you probably took this to mean was that the car would consistently do what you wanted it to do (start when you turn the key, slow down when you push the brakes). Reliability in assessment tools is broadly the same – you want the assessment tool to perform consistently. However, it is a little more complex than that and is often split into two types.

Intra-rater reliability relates to the consistency of the tool when used over and over again by the same person. Let's think back to Dean, the young man discussed at the start of the chapter. If the AUDIT and HADS tools used on Dean display good intra-rater reliability, then if a patient with exactly the same characteristics as Dean was in front of you the next day, you would get the same AUDIT and HADS result from any assessment. The level of intra-rater reliability can be measured in a number of ways, but the simplest is called *test–retest reliability testing*. This type of testing could involve giving a nurse the assessment tool and asking them to use it for a sample patient. The nurse is then asked to complete the tool a few weeks later for exactly the same patient – if the intra-reliability is good, then the nurse should get the same score each time.

Inter-rater reliability refers to the consistency of the assessment tools when used by different people. This can be quite difficult to ensure, as we all have very different ways of looking at the world. Generally speaking, if an assessment tool asks for our opinions – that is, if it is very subjective – then inter-rater reliability is low. If, on the other hand, questions are asked about concrete facts – if it is objective – then reliability is improved.

Let's take an example from outside healthcare: if you ask a number of people whether a new film was any good or not, then you are likely to receive many different answers. This is a subjective question with poor inter-rater reliability. If you were to ask the audience what the film was called – an objective fact – then the reliability will be good and you should receive the same answer from most people.

When you are caring for patients in practice, inter-rater reliability is crucial. There is no value in having a tool which gives you one answer, and then gives your colleague a different answer even if the characteristics of the patient haven't changed. Because of this, any new tool should be tested for reliability. Research summary 6.1 shows how the inter-rater reliability of a well-known assessment tool can be tested. Read the summary, and then think about what the findings mean for practice.

RESEARCH SUMMARY 6.1

One hundred and ten qualified nurses were given a written patient scenario and asked to complete a Waterlow assessment scale to assess the patient's risk of developing a pressure ulcer. Once all the nurses had completed their Waterlow scales, the scores were compared against each other.

When the results were analysed, it was found that there was a wide variation in the scores given. The 'correct' Waterlow score for the patient was 18. However, only 13 of the 110 nurses (12 per cent) actually got this score. Of the other nurses, the scores given ranged from 11 up to 35.

There were a number of reasons for the poor inter-rater reliability. Some nurses made incorrect assumptions about the patient in the scenario; others did not follow the instructions accurately. In some cases, nurses who used the tool every day in practice did not know what all the clinical terms meant. For example, patients should be given 8 marks if they have **terminal cachexia**, but 30 per cent of the nurses in the study didn't know what this phrase meant.

Kelly J (2005) Inter-rater reliability and Waterlow's pressure ulcer risk assessment tool. *Nursing Standard* 19(32): 86–92

The study by Kelly (2005) shows how assessment tools can be unreliable sometimes, particularly if nurses are not clear on how to use them correctly. This could have serious implications in practice: if the risk of pressure ulcers is underestimated then the proper precautions (such as pressure-relieving mattresses) might not be put in place. If the risk is overestimated then precautions might be taken that aren't necessary.

Terminal cachexia is the muscle-wasting and weight loss associated with the end-of-life stage of some illnesses.

> ## STOP AND THINK
>
> Look again at the assessment tools used in your own clinical areas. Have you been taught how to use them? Have they got clear instructions printed on them? Do you understand all the clinical terms in the assessment tool?

We've taken care of reliability; the next thing to think about is validity. Validity refers to the degree to which the assessment tool measures what it is intended to. That might seem a bit vague, so we'll look at the different types of validity, which might make things a bit clearer.

First, we have *face validity*. This can be tested by giving the assessment tool to anybody – ideally someone who is not an expert in healthcare – and asking them whether or not they think that 'on the face of it' the tool measures what it is supposed to (Parahoo 2006). Let's say that you want to develop an assessment tool to find out if a patient is at risk of falls in their own home. Your first attempt includes three questions – whether the patient lives in a house with an odd or even number, what football team the patient supports, and whether or not they are vegetarian. If you showed this tool to a friend or relative with no nursing knowledge they would (hopefully) tell you that these questions did not 'on the face of it' have anything to do with risk of falls – in other words, the face validity is poor. If you went back to your friend with a new version of the tool – this time including questions on what type of house the patient lived in, whether they had a history of falls, and what flooring they had – then they would tell you that this was a lot better. This is a fairly extreme example, but it does demonstrate how simple face validity can be.

Face validity is often talked about as a type of *content validity*. Although content validity refers to much the same thing – whether a tool measures what it is supposed to – the way in which it is tested is slightly different. Unlike face validity, in which the opinion of pretty much anyone can be sought, content validity is based upon the judgement of experts. Once an assessment tool has been developed, it is viewed by clinical experts, who will decide whether the right questions are being asked in the right way. The expert panel will also look at whether the questions asked are based on relevant research. Once the tool has been viewed and adapted by many experts, the content validity will have been maximised.

> ## STOP AND THINK
>
> Have another look at those assessment tools that you have used in your own practice. Based on your clinical expertise and knowledge, what do you think about the questions that are asked in the tool? Are the questions based on research? Would you have asked anything different?
>
> Answering these questions means that you have carried out your own assessment of the content validity of the assessment tools.

Content validity is important in any assessment tool and is the first thing that should be tested when developing something new. Research summary 6.2 describes an example of how the content validity of an assessment tool can be measured. However, even in the very robust approach described in this example, there is still the potential for subjectivity in the professional opinions expressed. To try and understand the validity of an assessment tool in even more depth, it is also useful to think about *criterion-based validity*.

RESEARCH SUMMARY 6.2

A study sought to establish the content validity of an oral assessment tool used in the care of children and young people with cancer. The researchers sent copies of the assessment tool to 19 experts in this area of care – dentists, oncologists and paediatric oncology nurses – to gain their views on the tool itself and the different elements within it. As part of the assessment, each question within the tool was given a mark for relevance, and experts made suggestions for improvement.

The study found that most elements of the oral assessment tool were considered to be valid by the expert panel. However, the expert review did result in some changes being made: the order in which the assessment was carried out was altered and greater guidance on how to use the tool was inserted. One element of the assessment – pain description – was removed altogether as it was agreed that it may not always be a valid (or reliable) indicator of oral hygiene in children.

The research demonstrated how robust testing of content validity with expert panels can confirm the value of an assessment tool, whilst also helping to improve it further.

Gibson F, Cargill J, Allison J et al. (2006) Establishing content validity of the oral assessment guide in children and young people. *European Journal of Cancer* 42(12): 1817–1825

Criterion-based validity is tested by looking at how the findings of an assessment tool compare to other findings about the same patient. Just to try and confuse you a bit more, criterion-based validity can be further split into two types: concurrent and predictive (Parahoo 2006).

We'll start with an example of how concurrent criterion-based validity can be measured. Let's say that you were measuring a patient's level of pain using an assessment scale, and the scale suggests to you that the patient is suffering only mild pain. However, when you look at the patient, you see that they are writhing around the bed, clutching at their side, grimacing with agony. It is clear that your clinical observation of the patient tells you a very different story from the assessment scale: in other words, the concurrent validity of the scale seems to be poor.

The second type of criterion-based validity is predictive validity. As the name suggests, this relates to how good an assessment scale is at predicting future outcomes or behaviour. We've already talked about a number of assessment tools that are used to predict events such as falls, development of pressure ulcers or depression. To test the validity of these tools, we can look at what actually happened, to see if they accurately predicted it. If we had an assessment tool to predict someone's risk of becoming dependent on alcohol, then we could find out how many people actually did develop an alcohol problem to find out the accuracy of the prediction.

There are two more terms that we need to talk about – specificity and sensitivity. Again, these are terms that you might have heard of in relation to research, but they are also important for many assessment tools. First of all, sensitivity, not surprisingly, relates to how sensitive the tool is when it comes to predicting the future. It is obviously really important that an assessment tool has a high level of sensitivity – for example, if a patient is suffering from depression, then the tool needs to detect this. If someone is at risk of malnutrition, then the assessment tool is of little use if it fails to predict this. If a tool is not very sensitive, you often get what are referred to as 'false-negative' results. If you use a tool with low sensitivity you may, for example, be told that a patient is at very low risk of falling even if their true risk is very high. This obviously has serious implications for patient safety, as they may not get the care that they require to prevent problems occurring or to treat existing problems. Generally speaking then, we want to be sure that any tool we use is as close to being 100 per cent sensitive as possible.

Sensitivity, though, is only half the story. To try and demonstrate this, we'll make a prediction. *We predict that everyone who reads this book will, at some time in their life, need a hip replacement.* On the face of it, this may seem a ridiculous statement, as reading this book does not make you any more likely to need a new hip. Nevertheless, despite this, our prediction is 100 per cent sensitive. At some stage in their lives, a small number of people who have read this book will require a hip replacement, and we have accurately predicted this years in advance. The truth is, it is very easy to make a tool sensitive, but on its own this is of little use. With relation to the hip replacement prediction, although we may have been right for a small number of readers, the vast majority of you will not need a hip replacement, and we therefore predicted something that was not going to happen – this is sometimes referred to as a 'false-positive'. False-positives can be a problem: let's assume that, after using an assessment tool, you thought that a patient was at risk of developing a pressure sore. In response to this, you might use all sorts of resources – such as pressure-relieving mattresses – to prevent this, even if the patient is really at low risk. In addition, false-positives might cause the patient unnecessary concern, just like the worry you may be experiencing right now about your future need for a hip replacement.

To try and prevent false-positives, we also need a tool to have a high level of *specificity* – the level to which the tool focuses in on those individuals who really are at risk or already have a problem. The prediction that we made about hip replacements for all our readers had a very low level of specificity, because it made a sweeping statement about everybody. The best assessment tools manage to have a high level of specificity – if they say that a patient is at high risk of a problem, they probably are.

STOP AND THINK

Thinking again about the assessment tools that you use in practice. What problems would be the caused if they had a low level of sensitivity and suggested that patients were not at risk even if they were? What if they had a low level of specificity and predicted that patients were at risk when they were not?

There's just one more element to a good assessment tool that we need to consider. In addition to being reliable, valid, sensitive and specific, a tool that is going to be used in practice needs to be acceptable. Although this is an important element, it is also very straightforward: is the tool easy to use for carers and their patients? If you were asked to go and assess a patient's risk of falling, and the assessment tool was a 15-page document containing 200 questions, how would you feel about doing it? How would the patient feel about being subjected to such a long assessment? If you look at some of the best-known assessment tools – such as the Waterlow score, the HADS, the Barthel Index – you'll see that they are all fairly short and easy to use.

Just to sum up, then, any assessment tool needs to be reliable, valid and acceptable. In addition, those that are trying to diagnose or predict problems should be sensitive and specific. If they are properly tested and meet all these requirements, then they can provide the benefits discussed at the start of the chapter: they can help with you decision making, they allow you to target resources at the patients who need them most, and they give you a clear baseline of how the patient is.

STOP AND THINK

Have another think about the assessment tools that you use in practice. Are there any things that you don't like about using them? Do your colleagues have any negative thoughts about using assessment tools?

WHAT HAVE YOU LEARNT SO FAR?

+ Assessment tools must be properly tested before being introduced in practice.
+ Assessment tools should be reliable – working consistently when used by yourself and other colleagues on a number of occasions with different patients.
+ Assessment tools should be valid. They should ask the right questions to find out about the problem accurately.
+ Sensitivity and specificity are important characteristics of assessment tools.
+ Assessment tools must be acceptable for those using them and for patients.

Disadvantages of assessment tools

Despite the advantages that we've talked about, there are some problems with using assessment tools. The main problem is that there is a tendency for nurses to become too reliant on assessment tools. This really causes difficulty if the assessment tool is not reliable or valid. Practice example 6.3 gives an illustration of how putting too much faith in an assessment tool can cause problems.

Practice example 6.3

Mrs Padmore is an 83-year-old woman who lives at home alone. Following concerns from her family about her safety, Mrs Padmore is visited by a community nurse, who carries out a falls assessment using a tool that was written locally. This tool suggests that Mrs Padmore is at low risk of falls.

Because of the findings, the community nurse does not feel that Mrs Padmore needs any more assessment and believes that her home environment must be safe. Two weeks after the assessment, Mrs Padmore has one of her 'dizzy spells', falls over and fractures her hip.

By using the results from assessment tools as the only piece of evidence in your decision making about patients, you run the risk of mistakes being made. It's important to remember that any assessment tool – no matter how well tested – can be misused or give false results. Because of this, you should consider the findings of any assessment tool as just one part of the assessment jigsaw. The findings should *add* to your clinical decision-making skills, not replace them. In some cases – particularly those areas of care where you are experienced and knowledgeable – it may be that you do not always need to use an assessment tool at all. For example, Anthony *et al.* (2010) suggest that clinical judgement can be just as good at predicting pressure ulcer risk as those tools (Waterlow; Norton; Braden) we discussed earlier.

Using your own assessment skills – observation, questioning, listening, deducing – is also important for your own professional development. Your assessment skills are like muscles: if you don't use them, you lose them. Simply filling in assessment tools all day would eventually 'deskill' you, making your clinical assessment skills less and less effective. Although assessment tools will always be an important part of your assessment, never forget about using your own judgement and instinct to recognise any actual problems.

Another potential problem with using assessment tools for your patients is that they do not really encourage a particularly 'holistic' approach. Instead, each assessment tool simply focuses on one aspect of the patient. Using a range of assessment tools gives you lots of information about different parts of the patient, but you don't get the holistic overview that we really need. One way of overcoming this is to use a nursing model in the way that we discussed in Chapter 3. Let's take the Activities of Living Model (Roper, Logan and Tierney 2000) as an example. Part of that holistic assessment asks that we explore issues around how the patient maintains a safe environment – the Waterlow score or the STRATIFY falls assessment could therefore give some valuable information about this. Assessment tools could even help us to gain some information about the factors influencing each of the activities of living. In other words, assessment tools shouldn't be used *instead* of a holistic assessment, but as just one part of it.

Conclusion

We've covered a lot of ground in this chapter, so let's just go over the main points about assessment tools one more time. First of all, there are different types of assessment tools:

+ health screening and diagnostic (for example, HADS and AUDIT);
+ descriptive (such as the Barthel Index and pain assessment tools);
+ predictive (such as the Waterlow score and STRATIFY falls scale).

Any assessment tool that is used in practice should go through a number of tests to check that it is reliable, valid, sensitive and specific. Going through these tests makes sure that any information that you get from assessment tools really does reflect the condition of your patient.

If you use them properly, assessment tools can be incredibly useful. They can give you a reminder of what questions to ask or observations to make; they can give you a clear idea of a patient's diagnosis or level of risk; they can allow you to target equipment and treatment at those patients who most need it. However, there are also risks. Don't let yourself rely too much on assessment tools: they are there to help, not to replace your own clinical judgement and decision-making skills.

Further reading

We've spoken about some of the best-known assessment tools in this chapter. If you want to find out more about these specific tools, then some suggestions for further reading would be:

Alcohol misuse screening: Reinert D, Allen J (2007) The Alcohol Use Disorders Identification Test: an update of research findings. *Alcoholism: Clinical and Experimental Research* 31(2): 185–199.

Hospital Anxiety and Depression Scale: Bjelland I, Dahl A, Haug T *et al.* (2002) The validity of the Hospital Anxiety and Depression Scale. An updated literature review. *Journal of Psychosomatic Research* 52: 69–77.

Nutritional screening tools: Green S, Watson R (2006) Nutritional screening and assessment tools for older adults: literature review. *Journal of Advanced Nursing* 54: 477–490.

For a more general look at validity, reliability, measurement and much more, albeit from a research rather than assessment tool viewpoint, try:

Parahoo K (2006) *Nursing Research. Principles, Process and Issues,* 2nd ed. Basingstoke: Palgrave Macmillan.

Or:

Waltz C, Strickland O, Lenz E (2010) *Measurement in Nursing and Health research.* 4th ed. New York: Springer Publishing Company.

Chapter 7
Organising care planning and delivery

Why this chapter matters

Imagine that you've just carried out a comprehensive assessment of a 75-year-old woman called Mrs Perkins. During your assessment Mrs Perkins tells you that she is suffering with constipation. You therefore explore this problem in more detail, finding out, for example, how long it is since she last opened her bowels, what remedies she's tried, and whether she's suffered from constipation before. Once you've finished your assessment, you have to plan the care required to help manage Mrs Perkins' constipation. Do you . . .

1. Take a blank piece of paper and handwrite a plan of care?
2. Go to a filing cabinet and get a pre-printed care plan for patients with constipation?
3. Use a care pathway that tells you what to do about constipation and when to do it?
4. Type 'constipation' into a computer database and print out the appropriate care plan?
5. Not bother using a plan of care at all – after all, you know what you're doing, so why waste time on a load of paperwork?

Chapter 1 explained why option 5 is not appropriate: If you don't use a plan of care at all, then other members of the healthcare team won't know what you're doing, Mrs Perkins will not be able to read about her care, and there will be no records to refer to if a complaint is made. So, given that you *must* have a plan of care, which is the best sort to have?

This chapter looks at the different ways that care is documented in clinical practice. Broadly speaking, we'll look at two types of documentation – care plans and care pathways. These come in different shapes and sizes: some handwritten, some pre-printed and some electronic. Once you've read through the chapter, you'll know more about the strengths and weaknesses of documentation methods. You'll also see how different types of care planning are best suited to different patients in different clinical settings. By making sure that you use the right sort of documentation for each of your patients, you can make your own care planning even better.

By the end of this chapter you will be able to:

+ explain the differences between individualised care plans, core care plans and care pathways;

+ discuss the strengths and weaknesses of different types of care planning documentation.

Care plans

Care plans are the traditional way of documenting problems, writing goals for patients to achieve, and listing ways that the patient can be helped. Because care plans have been around for years, different ways of producing them have evolved. The first way we'll look at is probably the oldest version of care planning – starting with a completely blank piece of paper and writing (either by hand or on a computer) the care plan from scratch. Calling this the 'starting with a blank piece of paper and writing the care plan from scratch method' is a bit over the top, so we need another name. Because this approach requires you to write a new care plan for every patient, we'll call it 'individualised' care planning.

The first thing to say is that as a nurse, you should be able to write an individualised care plan. Even if you work in an area where individualised care plans are never used, it's still a skill you should possess. You should be able to sit down with a patient, assess their needs, diagnose their problems, write some goals and list the nursing care required – just like we talked about in Chapter 2. It's not just we who think this: as Chapter 1 explored, the Nursing and Midwifery Council – the professional body for registered nurses in the UK – includes care planning as a competency to be achieved by all those completing their pre-registration nursing programme (NMC 2010b).

So why is this skill so important? First, this is the only type of care planning that is completely focused on the patient as an individual. Unlike the methods discussed later in this chapter, there are no pre-printed sections, no preconceived goals and no tick-boxes. Like the blank canvas used by an artist, a blank piece of paper allows you to paint a unique picture of patient needs and nursing care. You could think of an individualised care plan as being like a tailored suit, based upon a person's own measurements and designed to fit absolutely perfectly. This 'bespoke' care planning should help your patients receive high-quality, individualised nursing interventions. In some research, nurses do indeed seem to think that individualised planning can benefit patient care (Björvell *et al.* 2003).

Aside from the possible benefits for patients, individualised care plans are also thought to be good for nursing as a profession. Because they are based on a comprehensive assessment, include a detailed plan and make reference to implementation and evaluation, they reflect all the stages of ASPIRE – the problem-solving approach to care discussed in Chapter 2. Individualised care plans could therefore be seen as a way for nurses to show, in writing, exactly how complex their job is. If a patient, visitor, manager or other healthcare worker asks the question 'What exactly do nurses do?', then a properly written care plan will give them all the information they need.

So far, so good: individualised care plans tell us exactly what care patients need and what we as nurses have to do. They also provide evidence of the problem-solving approach to nursing care, and therefore 'show off' the professional role to other people.

But . . . these strengths come at a cost. In particular, producing an individualised care plan from scratch takes up a lot of time. In one (admittedly fairly old) piece of research, Martin *et al.* (1999) found that some nurses needed to spend over a quarter of their working day simply trying to write and maintain patient care plans. In another study, Allen (1998) found that nurses lacked the time to read (let alone update) patient care plans. If there's not enough time to produce and maintain care plans, then they won't be as well-written or useful as they could be. Some nurse researchers have found that nurses cut corners to save time when using individualised care plans: some are written *after* care has been given, rather than planning care in advance; some care plans are written without considering patients' individual needs; some are just left unfinished (Cheevakasemsook *et al.* 2006; Mason 1999).

Another weakness is that there is no overwhelming evidence that writing and maintaining an individualised care plan actually improves nursing practice or helps patients recover any more quickly. Research summary 7.1 provides just one demonstration of this point. The lack of evidence is a big problem. Everything that we do in nursing – from different ways of administering injections through to determining how long patients are kept 'nil by mouth' before operations – should be based on evidence that it works. If there is no evidence that individualised care plans improve care, then what is the point of us spending time writing them? This negative view of individualised care plans is widespread in practice. Nurses often feel that individualised care plans are a 'paper exercise', needlessly taking up time that they could spend actually giving hands-on patient care (Cheevakasemsook *et al.* 2006).

RESEARCH SUMMARY 7.1

Urquhart and colleagues carried out a Cochrane review of the effects on outcomes of different nursing record systems. A Cochrane review is a high-quality, structured review of the evidence base for a specific topic area (much more information and all the reviews can be found at www.cochrane.org/cochrane-reviews).

They reviewed a total of nine studies (eight randomised controlled trials and one before-and-after study). The review found that when nursing records were focused on discrete and specific problems (e.g. pain relief in children), they seemed to improve care and outcomes. However, benefits were more uncertain in those studies that looked at broader nurse care planning systems.

Urquhart C, Currell R, Grant MJ, Hardiker NR (2009) Nursing record systems: effects on nursing practice and health care outcomes. *Cochrane Database of Systematic Reviews* 2009 (1).

Before we look at alternatives to individualised care plans, we'll just say a couple of things in their defence. First of all, although there is no evidence that they improve patient care, there is also no research that suggests individual care plans have any detrimental effects on the care given to patients. We should also think about how the standard of nursing care is measured in research. A lot of studies measure the standard of care through patient outcomes, such as the length of time spent in hospital. There is, however, very little research looking at the impact of individualised care plans on areas such as patient satisfaction, communication, and the relationship between the nurse and their patient – areas where individualised care plans might make a difference.

STOP AND THINK

Have you ever produced an individualised care plan for patients in your care? Did you have enough time to do it properly? Do you think it improved patient care? Do you think it is a practical method of care planning for your current place of work?

Whether you're a fan of individualised care plans or not, there is no getting away from one fact: they do take a lot of time to write and maintain. Given that time is something in short supply during any nurse's day, it is no surprise that alternatives to individualised care plans have become popular in healthcare. The first of these alternative methods is based on the fact that different patients often have very similar problems. Practice example 7.1 provides a description of a situation where two patients have similar needs.

Instances such as that described in Practice example 7.1 have led to the widespread use of standardised, prewritten care plans. These types of care plan were described by Walsh (1994) as 'core' care plans, and we'll stick with that name for the rest of the book. Core care plans are the 'off-the-peg' alternative to the tailored version. They include a number of pre-written problems, goals and nursing interventions linked to a specific issue. Have a look at Activity 7.1.

Practice example 7.1

Melanie is a community nurse who has, amongst her caseload, two patients with similar problems. Mrs Smith and Mrs Green are both widows in their eighties, and are both housebound.

Both patients have urinary catheters *in situ* due to problems with incontinence, and both have leg ulcers. Rather than writing completely new care plans for both patients, Melanie recognises that elements of care for both patients will be the same. The community nursing team has developed a range of standardised, prewritten care plans that contain need statements, goals and nursing interventions. From this collection of care plans, Melanie selects those written for the care of patients with urinary catheters and leg ulcer management.

Activity 7.1

Think about the patients you care for at work. Can you list five patient problems that you commonly have to deal with (e.g. constipation)?

Take one of those problems and write down some common interventions that you would use to deal with this issue (e.g. encourage high-fibre diet).

If you've had a go at Activity 7.1, then, effectively, you've started to write a core care plan. The most obvious advantage of core care plans, when compared with individualised care plans, is that you don't have to write every element of care from scratch, so precious time is saved. In the case of Practice example 7.1, Melanie can go to a filing cabinet or onto a computer, get core care plans for urinary catheters and leg ulcers, and put these into the patient notes. By doing so, the patients have documentation related to their problems, and you have saved yourself a significant amount of time. The time saved by using core care plans can then be spent providing direct patient care (Lee and Chang 2004; O'Connell *et al.* 2000).

As well as the time benefits, the use of core care plans should mean that all patients with the same problem will receive consistent nursing care. Core care plans should also be written in line with the very latest guidance and research related to that problem and updated if any new evidence is found. The result of this is that core care plans should promote standardised, evidence-based care for all patients (O'Connell *et al.* 2000). One final (and very practical) advantage of core care plans is that, because they are printed, nurses don't have to struggle to read each other's messy handwriting (Lee and Chang 2004)!

The key weakness of core care plans is that they don't automatically take into account the individual needs of patients. Because they are written for *everybody* with a particular problem, the goals and interventions have to be very general, providing a 'best fit' for the majority of patients. If we go back to the suit analogy, then although the 'off-the-peg' choice will fit most people fairly well, it may not be suitable for people who are an unusual shape or who have individual preferences such as a particular type of button or size of pockets. Similarly, patients under your care – even if they have the same broad problem – will all have different reactions to their problems, different preferences for care and different fears.

Take the patients in Practice example 7.1: although Mrs Green and Mrs Smith both have leg ulcers and urinary catheters, their actual needs may be very different. Mrs Smith may be capable of managing her urinary catheter by herself, and may not be concerned by the leg ulcer, which seems to be healing well. Mrs Green, however, may require more help with her catheter and may be very upset by a leg ulcer that is leaking foul-smelling discharge and appears to be getting worse. Simply using identical core care plans for both patients would not recognise the huge differences between Mrs Smith and Mrs Green. To overcome this problem, it is crucial that Melanie uses the core care plans as a broad template, but then adapts each plan to each patient's individual needs. For example, although the core care plan may state that patients with leg ulcers need dressings changing every six to seven days, Mrs Green may need hers changing every other day until it begins to heal.

It is generally accepted that to be effective, core care plans should be adapted in response to individual patient needs (Walsh 1994). However, this is not always done as well as it should be. In some areas, the only change made to core care plans is filling in a blank space with the patient's name. For example '_____ is complaining of postoperative nausea and vomiting'. In one study, Mason (1999) found that a core care plan for patient anxiety was being used for all 20 patients on one ward. However, no adaptations had been made to any of the care plans, other than writing in each individual patient's name. Each of those 20 patients may indeed have been anxious, but the *reasons* for their anxiety may have been entirely different.

Practice example 7.2 shows how patients can have fears and anxieties that are individual to them. It gives an example of why, even when using core care plans, it is so important to carry out a really detailed assessment. In Deidre's case it was not simply enough to know that she was anxious – it was crucial for the nurse to find out the *cause* of the anxiety. The other important part of Practice example 7.2 is that the nurse adapted the care plan to meet Deidre's individual needs.

Practice example 7.2

Ward 7 is a surgical ward that uses core care plans. One care plan, used for preoperative anxiety, is placed in the nursing notes of all patients. The care plan states that anxiety should be reduced, and it provides a range of interventions to achieve this, including showing patients around the ward and providing them with information leaflets.

Deidre is a 68-year-old woman, admitted for an elective surgical procedure. The core care plan for anxiety is included within her nursing documentation. Deidre is extremely anxious, but not because of the impending surgery. Instead, Deidre is terrified of lifts and knows that she will need to be transported to and from the operating theatre via the patient transport lifts.

Fortunately, the nurse caring for Deidre has carried out a comprehensive assessment of the factors that are causing her anxiety. This has allowed the nursing team to recognise the fear of lifts and individualise the core care plan accordingly. As a result, negotiations with the surgical team have led to an agreement that Deidre can be transferred to a ward on the same floor as theatres, thereby removing the need for travelling in the lifts.

Summarising the strengths and weaknesses of core care plans is fairly easy to do. They do save time in comparison with individualised care plans, and therefore they let you spend more of your working day actually looking after patients. However, if they're not used properly, then they become a rather pointless part of the nursing notes. Patients should still be assessed properly (see Chapters 2 and 8) and their individual needs diagnosed. Once this has been done, core care plans can be used as the framework for planning, but they should then be adapted so that they meet the specific needs of your patients.

STOP AND THINK

Do you use core care plans in your own clinical area? Do you find them useful? Are they written in such a way that you can adapt the goals and interventions for each patient? Do you think that they are adapted enough in practice?

So far, we've looked at individualised and core care plans. Both approaches have strengths and weaknesses: individualised care plans are time-consuming but reflect the individual needs of patients; core care plans save time, but do not always account for differences between patients. Some nurses dislike both types of care plan, and question whether they serve any purpose nowadays. These criticisms are mainly due to problems with the way care plans are used – they are often incomplete and inaccurate, they rarely include the patient's thoughts and feelings, and they are not produced to a consistent standard (Cheevakasemsook *et al.* 2006). Others fail to see the point of spending time on care plans when there is no evidence that they actually improve the care given.

Fortunately, for those nurses who view care plans as outdated, irrelevant and unhelpful, there is another way. In the 1980s, an alternative form of care documentation was developed in the USA. This new type of documentation was called – amongst other things – a care pathway, and it has quickly become a hugely popular alternative to the more traditional care plan.

Care pathways

Care pathways are known by lots of different names, such as integrated care pathways, anticipated recovery paths and care maps (Campbell *et al*. 1998), but we'll stick with 'care pathways' for the rest of the book. They were first developed in the USA as one element of an approach to healthcare called 'managed care' – a system that tries to cut costs and improve the quality of care (Hale *et al*. 1999; Riley 1998).

Care pathways tend to have a number of common characteristics. First, they are multidisciplinary in nature, meaning that they are written, used and updated by all members of the healthcare team (which is why they are sometimes called 'integrated' care pathways). Secondly, care pathways are usually produced for a specific group of patients. For example, a care pathway might be written for patients undergoing tonsillectomy, or patients suffering from dementia. Finally, care pathways include a list of things that need to be done for patients, and goals that patients should meet, set within a period of time (Hale *et al*. 1999).

Think of care pathways as being like route planners for car journeys. They both start at point A and finish at point B: on a route planner, this might be from Hull to Cardiff; in a care pathway, it could be from admission for **hysterectomy** through to discharge home. Route planners have a list of instructions (e.g. 'Join M1 at junction 32 and head south'), and so do care pathways (e.g. 'Give mouth care every hour'). These instructions are often known as 'processes' and are a crucial part of care pathways. In addition to processes, route planners also give you an idea of where you should be at different times of your journey – this gives you a rough idea of how long the journey should take and whether you are on schedule. Similarly, care pathways often include a list of goals that the patient should meet (e.g. 'To be pain-free on return from the operating theatre'). These progress points are called 'outcomes'. Most care pathways include a mixture of process and outcome so that the patient and healthcare team know what care is required, and when the patient should achieve certain goals in their recovery.

Of course, any car journey can be complicated by unexpected events. Roadworks can cause traffic jams, cars can have punctures, and children in the back can be sick all over themselves and the floor. Whenever these things happen, we alter the route plan to adapt to the new situation – taking a diversion, changing a tyre, or stopping to wash vomit off everything. Healthcare is equally unpredictable. For example, patients may not recover as quickly as anticipated, they may deteriorate unexpectedly, or they may decide to refuse the treatment prescribed in the care pathway.

Hysterectomy is surgical removal of the womb.

Crucially, care pathways offer healthcare practitioners a way of adapting to these individual needs and progress of patients. In a process known as variance monitoring, practitioners write down any changes from the processes or outcomes listed within the pathway. Practice example 7.3 provides an outline of how variance monitoring can be used in practice.

Practice example 7.3

Brian is a 56-year-old man admitted to a coronary care unit following a myocardial infarction (MI). He meets the criteria for the MI care pathway and has followed it since admission.

Because of the risk of abnormal heart rhythms following a MI, Brian has been on a heart monitor since admission. According to the care pathway, Brian should be removed from the cardiac monitor and be allowed to walk gently around the bed area on day 2 following his MI. However, Brian has had some abnormal heart rhythms since admission, so the multidisciplinary team has decided that he should remain on the heart monitor for at least another 24 hours. This decision is written in the variance monitoring section of the care pathway and reviewed 24 hours later.

Care pathways have been introduced throughout healthcare for a wide range of patient needs. These include short-term hospital-based care such as hip replacement, through to long-term community-based management of conditions such as heart failure (Bandolier 2003). Most care pathways have been written by individual healthcare organisations (e.g. National Health Service [NHS] trusts) for use in that setting alone. Some pathways are not just used within single organisations but have been introduced throughout the country. The best known example of this is the Liverpool Care Pathway for the Dying Patient (LCP), developed in the late 1990s. The LCP has quickly moved from being a document that was trialled on a local basis to one that is used nationwide. Since its introduction, the LCP has helped hospital and community services to work together more effectively, so that they can provide better care for dying patients (Ellershaw and Murphy 2005).

The popularity of care pathways such as the LCP reflects the fact that they have a number of advantages over traditional care plans. First, because most care pathways are multidisciplinary, there is no longer any need for separate notes written by nurses, doctors, physiotherapists, dieticians and other practitioners. Instead, one document includes all the necessary information about the patient, their progress and the care that they require. Because of this, communication is improved between professional groups, with no need to go searching different documents for entries from practitioners. It is also suggested that getting different healthcare professionals together to write a care pathway in the first place might improve working relationships (Walsh 1997). From the patients' point of view, shared documentation may also reduce the number of times that they are asked the same questions by different professionals.

In addition to improving communication between healthcare workers, the actual development of a care pathway is important for other reasons. To write a care pathway, the first thing that needs to be done is to choose a topic area. Let's assume that a group of clinicians is going to write a care pathway for patients diagnosed with hypertension (high blood pressure). Once the topic is agreed, a group of multidisciplinary healthcare professionals need to sit down and look at the latest research and guidelines related to that topic area (Campbell *et al*. 1998). In this case they would look at the latest evidence from journals, guidelines from professional bodies (such as the British Hypertension Society), and advice from organisations such as the National Institute for Health and Clinical Excellence (NICE). Once the group has agreed on what best practice is, they compare this with the care that they currently provide for patients with hypertension. This means that, by developing a care pathway, the group does not simply write down what already happens but actually changes the care that it provides to meet with the latest guidelines.

Once a care pathway is actually written, it will be continuously updated to make sure that it represents best practice and the needs of patients. The updating of care pathways happens because of the process of variance monitoring that was discussed earlier. Remember Brian in Practice example 7.3? When he was kept on the heart monitor for an extra day, this change from the plan would have been documented in the variance monitoring section of the care pathway. Once he was discharged home, his care pathway would have been reviewed and any variances would have been entered on to a computer database, along with all the other variances from every other patient who was on the MI care pathway. Every so often, the variances from care pathways will be reviewed by members of the multidisciplinary team. Let's imagine that the review of variances for the MI pathway showed that, in three-quarters of patients, removal from the heart monitor was – as in Brian's case – delayed because of abnormal heart rhythms. This might lead the multidisciplinary group who maintain the care pathway to make changes to the document, such as altering the suggested date of removal from monitoring. A pathway should therefore not be written and then left alone for years: it should be audited, discussed and changed to take account of patient needs and new evidence (De Luc 2000).

We've talked a bit about what care pathways are, how they are written and how they can be updated. The next thing to look at is whether or not they are useful to nurses and beneficial to patients. For student nurses, or those who have not been qualified very long, care pathways are very useful because they contain clear instructions on what care to provide. By giving step-by-step guidance on what to do, and what the patient should be doing, care pathways therefore support less experienced practitioners. Nurses with a greater level of expertise may not rely so heavily on the pathway to tell them what to do, but they are able to use their nursing knowledge and decision-making ability by recognising and acting upon variances (Gunstone and Robinson 2006).

As we saw earlier in the chapter, there does not seem to be any conclusive evidence that care plans actually improve the standard of care given to patients. In the case of care pathways, there is some better news. There have been a number of studies where the introduction of care pathways has been linked to reduced costs and decreased length of hospital stay (Dy *et al*. 2005; Ilag *et al*. 2003). Some research also suggests that using care pathways helps healthcare practitioners to follow evidence-based guidelines (Ilag *et al*. 2003) and may even aid patient recovery (Bandolier 2003). Overall, it seems that care pathways, if used correctly, can deliver a higher quality of care at a lower cost.

RESEARCH SUMMARY 7.2

We've already discussed the value of Cochrane reviews in this chapter. They provide a high-quality overview of the effectiveness of specific healthcare interventions. In 2010, Rotter and colleagues published a review of the effectiveness of care pathways on practice and outcomes.

They analysed findings from 27 studies that included a total of over 11,000 patients and compared usual care to care delivered under the guidance of a pathway. They found that care pathways could improve documentation and reduce in-hospital complications. Many of the studies included also demonstrated a reduction in length of stay. The authors concluded that pathways therefore bring benefits in terms of effective record keeping and in relation to key outcomes of care.

Rotter T, Kinsman L, James EL, *et al.* (2010) Clinical pathways: effects on professional practice, patient outcomes, length of stay and hospital costs. *Cochrane Database of Systematic Reviews:* 2010 (3)

If we accept that care pathways could help nurses and their patients, is the traditional care plan – and the problem-solving approach related to it – no longer required? Some nursing writers seem to think so: Walsh (1997) includes a subheading in his article on care pathways that reads 'Critical pathways: an alternative to the nursing process'. This suggests that care pathways can be used without a problem-solving approach to nursing, but we would have to disagree with this. Our view is that for care pathways to be of maximum use to nurses and their patients, the use of a problem-solving approach to care planning is absolutely vital.

Take the concept of variance monitoring that we discussed earlier in the chapter – how could a nurse tell that a patient has not met the outcomes within a care pathway without carrying out an in-depth assessment and then rechecking and evaluating the care given? Once a variance has been noted, how is it possible for you to plan effectively the care that deals with the variance without a problem-solving approach to the problem?

To emphasise the role of the problem-solving approach within care pathways it is important to look again at the purpose of variance monitoring. The use of the word 'monitoring' suggests that users of the care pathway simply make a note of any variances that occur. If you remember from earlier, the recording and monitoring of variances does have an important role in keeping pathways up-to-date and relevant. However, variances are much more important than this. If a patient does not get the treatment that is prescribed, or if they do not meet an expected goal, then something needs to be done about it. Once you recognise that a variance has occurred, the patient should be assessed to find out why there has been a deviation from the care pathway. You then need to work out how to manage the variance by setting goals and deciding upon nursing interventions. In essence, you should produce a 'micro' care plan for each variance that occurs. Maybe a change of name would help – rather than 'variance monitoring', let's call it 'variance management'. This name still recognises the need for variances to be recorded and reviewed, but it also reinforces the need for something to be done about them immediately, using a problem-solving approach to care.

Care pathways are here to stay. There is plenty of research suggesting that writing, using and updating care pathways can lower the cost of healthcare and may even improve the quality of care provided to patients. Because they will be an important part of healthcare, it is really important that you as a nurse are able to use them properly. Whenever variances from the pathway occur, nurses should recognise them and act upon them. For each variance, a 'micro' care plan should be produced using a problem-solving approach. By doing so, you can get the best out of care pathways, whilst also demonstrating the skills necessary to provide top-quality nursing care.

> **STOP AND THINK**
>
> Have you ever used a care pathway? If so, did you find it easy to follow? Was it easy to recognise variances from the expected patient progress? Do you think that care pathways meet the individual needs of your patients?

Electronic care plans

Information technology (IT) is everywhere, and we rely on it for many things that we do. This book is being written on a computer, it will be sent to the publisher by email, and it will (we hope) be bought by many people over the internet. Given that computers have an influence on almost every aspect of our lives, that we can use the internet to find out about anything, and that email allows us to share information incredibly easily, it is no surprise that IT now plays a huge role in healthcare.

The next time you're at work, think about the role played by IT. Wherever you work, the chances are that you will have access to a computer. This will probably allow you to access clinical results and may store images such as X-rays. Clinic appointments are often booked online nowadays, and some types of IT, such as tablet computers, are increasingly being used to assist nurses in specific clinical tasks such as the administration of medicines.

Lee (2006) describes how Electronic Patient Records (EPRs) have a number of benefits, such as allowing information to be accessed quickly, speeding up referrals to other practitioners, and helping nurses develop IT skills. However, there are – as with all care planning systems – still limitations. For example, it has been found that the time taken to update EPRs can detract from the time actually spent providing hands-on patient care (Laitinen et al. 2010).

Already, most care planning requires IT to be used. At a simple level, a core care plan or critical care pathway will have been written on a computer, so the content can be updated easily when necessary. In more sophisticated systems, a database of nursing diagnoses, goals and interventions is held on file and selected by nurses following assessment (Lee 2006).

> **STOP AND THINK**
>
> Think about the use of IT in your own clinical area. How big a part do computers play in the planning of care? Could they do more? Have you faced any problems when using computers in care planning?

Your role in the future of care planning

So, in a world of core care plans and care pathways, are individualised care plans no longer of any use? Are they are a relic of nursing's past, along with ridiculously frilly hats and salt baths? In many areas of clinical practice, the answer is – unfortunately – yes. Some writers now view the individualised nursing care plan as being of little practical use, existing only to promote the profession by providing written evidence of the nursing process having taken place (Allen 1998). Lee and Chang (2004) write about how care planning has 'developed' from being handwritten on blank sheets of paper, to being pre-printed according to set structures. Walsh (1998) describes individualised care plans as being part of a 'discredited' approach that does not automatically result in individualised care being provided. Many nurses we speak to tell us that individualised care plans seem to have largely disappeared from practice. Every time we teach individualised care planning to our pre-registration student nurses, we are met with a chorus of 'Why do we need to learn this? It never happens in practice.'

From this evidence, you might think that the future of care planning does not include individualised plans written from scratch. However, when you read the next few chapters of this book, you'll quickly notice that a lot of the discussion is about *how* to write an individualised care plan. Why? Are we – the authors – cynical old nurses who wistfully look back at the good old days of individualised care planning through rose-tinted spectacles? Well, yes, but that's not the point: the reason that this book teaches you how to produce an individualised care plan is because it is a skill that all nurses should possess, for a number of reasons.

First, individualised care planning still takes place in some settings. Those areas where the nurse–patient relationship has the time to be nurtured on a one-to-one basis, such as in the community setting, still use individualised care plans. Secondly, to be able to use the types of documentation that will be most common in the future – core care plans and care pathways – you still need the skill to write and use an individualised care plan. As we discussed earlier in the chapter, core care plans need to be adapted to meet the needs of individual patients, and variances from care pathways need 'micro' care plans to deal with them – these tasks need nurses to use care planning skills. Some patients will have problems for which core care plans or care pathways have not been written, and they will need individual care plans. Finally, core care plans and care pathways need writing in the first place; only someone with very well-developed care planning skills will be able to do this.

It is for these reasons that the rest of this book focuses on the steps that should be taken to plan care on an individual patient-by-patient basis, rather than simply describing how to follow a core care plan or clinical pathway. Think of reading and understanding the rest of the book as being like learning to drive a car with a manual gearbox. Once you have done this, you will be able to drive either a manual or an automatic car. On the other hand, if you only learn to drive in an automatic, you won't be able to operate a manual gearbox. In other words, an ability to write an individual care plan on a blank piece of paper will give you the skills that you need to use any type of nursing documentation. However, if you only know how to follow a core care plan or care pathway, then you won't have the skills to individualise care when you need to.

In the future, plans of patient care will certainly look very different from how they look today. There will be greater and greater use of electronic care plans. Most documentation will be in the form of core care plans and care pathways, and there will be greater emphasis on multidisciplinary plans of care. However, despite all these changes, you will still need to be able to demonstrate a skill that the Nursing and Midwifery Council says is a core part of the role: to be able to formulate and document a plan of nursing care (NMC 2010b).

Conclusion

Let's just recap the main points that we've covered in this chapter. Care planning can be organised in three main ways:

+ **Individualised care plans:** provide documentation that is tailored precisely to fit the patient's needs. They do take a long time to write and update, and they are used less and less in practice.

+ **Core care plans:** include goals and interventions for problems that many patients may have. They save a lot of time when compared with individualised care plans, but if they are not adapted for each patient's needs, then they may not be very useful.

+ **Care pathways:** written for specific diseases or procedures, and provide a timeline of care, with a mixture of interventions (process) and expected progress (outcomes). There is evidence that using care pathways can reduce healthcare costs and improve the quality of care. However, to ensure that care is individualised, nurses must use their care-planning skills to identify and manage variances from the expected pathway.

Whatever the form of documentation used, you must be competent in the use of a problem-solving approach to care planning. The next section of this book explores an approach that can be used by all nurses when planning care.

Further reading

Lee T (2006) Nurses' perceptions of their documentation experiences in a computerized nursing care planning system. *Journal of Clinical Nursing* 15: 1376–1382.

www.library.nhs.uk/pathways/ – holds copies of care pathways used within the NHS. If you are interested in finding out which care pathways already exist, then this is a very useful place to start.

www.connectingforhealth.nhs.uk – provides an overview of the development of electronic record keeping and information systems within the NHS.

For a practical introduction to care pathways, an interesting textbook, though a little dated, is:

Middleton S, Roberts E (2000) *Integrated Care Pathways: A Practical Approach to Implementation.* Edinburgh: Butterworth Heinemann.

Part 2
Application to practice

Chapter 8
Assessment

Why this chapter matters

The whole purpose of a nursing model is to guide your practice; it is meant to offer a framework to help you through the stages of the problem-solving approach. In the words of Aggleton and Chalmers (2000, p. 17), nursing models will 'help those who use them to understand more fully what they are doing and why they are doing it'.

Since we have outlined the beliefs and values of the three models, we now need to consider how the philosophy of each model is used alongside the problem-solving approach, by describing and exploring how the theories direct the stages of ASPIRE. We will be making use of the three scenarios in the appendices to illustrate how you can use the appropriate model and ASPIRE to create safe, effective care plans for your patients. In this chapter we will concentrate on the first stage of the ASPIRE approach – assessment.

By the end of the chapter, you will be able to:

+ conduct an assessment using Roper, Logan and Tierney's Activities of Living Model, Orem's Self-Care Model of Nursing and the Neuman Systems Model;
+ list the strengths and limitations of using these frameworks to assess patients' needs.

Assessment using the Activities of Living Model

Roper, Logan and Tierney (2000) prefer to use the word 'assessing' rather than 'assessment' because they suggest that assessment is an ongoing, active process, not a one-off task. The aims of assessing when using RLT are to:

+ collect information;
+ review and order the information;
+ identify the problems;
+ prioritise the problems.

Each of the 12 activities of living is considered in order to identify:

+ previous routines – how patients normally carry out the activities of living;
+ present routines – how they are carrying out the activities now.

If there is a difference between the previous and present ability to carry out an activity of living that demonstrates movement along the dependence–independence continuum (making the patient more dependent), the assessment continues. If there is no difference between the patient's previous and present routines, then you record the information as a baseline of their position on the dependence–independence continuum, but there is no need to explore this activity of living further.

The need to carry out an assessment such as this means that you need to establish a therapeutic relationship with your patient as soon as you are able – a task that involves talking, but most importantly observing and listening. To find out if there has been any movement along the dependence–independence continuum, it is important that you ask appropriate questions to establish how they usually carry out the activity and how they are carrying it out now – or, in other words, what they could do and what they can do now. From this you will be able to establish their normal position on the dependence–independence continuum and whether there has been any movement. If there has been movement you will not only identify the actual problem but also gain a sense of how 'big' the problem is. Sometimes you may find that it is unnecessary to explore all 12 activities of living, although Newton (1991) argues that all the activities should be considered and taken into account in order to make the assessment holistic and comprehensive.

It is also important to establish coping strategies, or ways in which patients deal with their problem; this will include adaptive and maladaptive strategies (ways that help and ways that make things worse). The philosophy of RLT's model is to promote independence; therefore, it is crucial to find out how the patient is coping with the change in dependence. If the coping strategy is a productive or adaptive one that helps the patient carry out the activity by dealing with the problem, then it needs to be encouraged and extended. Wherever possible, nursing actions should be organised around the patient's current ways of dealing with the activities of living and seek to build upon these routines, if they are adaptive. This is partly because it is often easier to modify an existing behaviour than substitute a new one, but also because patients are more likely to follow the plan of care if it is individualised to their needs and ways of carrying out their activities of living. Don't forget, though, that consideration of the coping strategies should not be limited to the physical ways of dealing with problems; it is just as important to consider the psychological, sociocultural and spiritual ways of coping. One last thing to say is that sometimes the decision as to whether a coping strategy is adaptive or not depends on whose point of view you are considering. A patient may choose to smoke because they feel it helps them deal with their stress, so for them it is adaptive. As a healthcare professional you will see that this is not, in the long term, an adaptive way of coping with stress.

Your assessment of the patient should also consider any influencing factors – the reasons behind the movement along the dependence–independence continuum. Remember, there are five categories that need to be considered – biological, sociocultural, psychological, environmental and politicoeconomic. Sometimes the patients will be able to tell you what the influencing factors are, but at other times the answer will come from laboratory reports, other healthcare professionals or your own clinical knowledge and judgements.

Consideration of the input of others – family, friends, carers or other healthcare providers – is relevant to the assessment. The overriding message of the RLT philosophy is to promote independence. This means that you need to be mindful not to step in and perform the activities unless you really have to; therefore, it makes sense to identify the input of friends and family as their actions may be ensuring that the activities are performed.

There is also a need to identify the interventions and treatments prescribed or carried out by others, e.g. doctors, physiotherapists, occupational therapists or counsellors, because there may be nursing care that arises from their interventions. An example of this may be when a doctor has prescribed a pain-relieving medication such as morphine. This intervention will call for nursing care in terms of giving the medication and monitoring for side effects, but the prescription also affects the patient's ability to carry out the activity of eliminating because constipation may occur as a result of giving an opiate. You will then have to offer nursing care to deal with the potential problem of constipation.

To provide some structure to assessment, RLT suggest a two-stage approach.

First stage

The first stage of assessment involves you confirming information about the patient in order to create a baseline that can be used later in the process. This information might include:

+ biographical information (such as name, age, address, next of kin);
+ health information (such as previous medical history and current medication).

Second stage

The second stage explores the patient's ability to carry out each activity of living (AL). If you follow these steps, you will change your focus from 'problem listing' to a process that produces a holistic, comprehensive assessment. Carrying out the second stage involves a number of actions on your part. You need to:

+ establish the patient's previous routine and describe how they usually carry out the AL, including where they are on the dependence–independence continuum normally
+ establish the patient's present routine or ability to carry out the AL, including where they are on the dependence–independence continuum now;
+ consider their coping strategies and any help that they have in carrying out the AL from family, friends or carers;
+ identify the influencing factors or the causes of movement along the dependence–independence continuum;
+ identify the nursing care that arises from any interventions/treatments prescribed or carried out by others.

Once you have conducted the assessment process you will need to categorise the information under the appropriate AL. This doesn't mean that the ALs should be used as a checklist to ask patients how they feel about communicating, expressing sexuality or dying. Whilst the ALs can serve as a prompt to help you remember the complexity of an individual's life, the conversation between you and your patient should be as natural as possible. Listen to your patient; let them disclose their experiences of carrying out the ALs so that you can identify the problems together. Understanding the assessment process will offer you a 'prompt' or structure to help steer the conversation around to establishing their normal routines, present routines, influencing factors, coping strategies and whether there is nursing care that arises from any interventions/treatments prescribed or carried out by others.

The model offers a 'conceptual framework' for you to conduct a holistic assessment. It is meant to guide you, not create rigid parameters that restrict the process. Remember, the ALs are meant to represent the activity in its broadest sense, as discussed in Chapter 3. Your patient is an individual so it is impossible to have a set of questions or list of 'typical responses' that need to be addressed under the heading of each AL. Gather all your information following the assessment stages and then decide which of the ALs the information should be categorised under.

In collaborative working, a full detailed account is necessary to allow everyone access to an accurate picture of the patient's needs (present and near future) and how they are affecting their ability to carry out the ALs. The assessment should offer a description of where the patient is on the dependence–independence continuum and what factors have contributed to their position; this information should, in turn, be set against the 'normal routine' for that patient.

The information gathered and categorised under the headings should facilitate the discovery of actual and potential problems, the identification of need statements and baselines, the setting of goals and the establishing of available resources to meet these goals. This suggests that a thorough assessment is one that provides information that makes the next stages of care planning much easier to carry out. The problem is that, if the assessment process is not adhered to or is not as thorough as it should be, then the next stages will be difficult and reflect the shortfalls of the procedure.

Have a look at Activity 8.1.

Activity 8.1

Safeedah is a 50-year-old woman who has recently been diagnosed with cancer of the breast. Originally from India, she has lived in England for three years and has come into the hospital in order to undergo a **mastectomy** and a course of **radiotherapy**.

The assessment made by the nurse (with the help of an interpreter) used RLT's Activities of Living Model and was as follows:

+ **Communicating** – wears glasses, cannot speak English.
+ **Expressing sexuality** – likes to wear make-up and dresses in a feminine way.
+ **Dying** – not discussed.

Think about the two-stage assessment process that RLT suggest and try to identify the strengths and limitations of the attempt.

Mastectomy is the surgical removal of a breast.

Radiotherapy is treatment of cancer through the use of radiation.

Overall, the practitioner's attempt in Activity 8.1 doesn't really offer an assessment of Safeedah's individual needs. The account concentrates on listing problems rather than exploring how she carries out the activity of living in her own unique way. There is no real evidence to suggest that the assessment used the two-stage process to establish Safeedah's previous routine, present routine, influencing factors, her coping strategies or the nursing care arising from any interventions/treatments prescribed or carried out by others. There is also a requirement to consider the needs that arise as the individual moves along the developmental lifespan continuum. It is necessary to acknowledge that developmental needs do not refer just to the demands that arise from the physical changes that accompany maturity. It is equally important to consider the psychological and sociocultural needs that arise as the individual progresses along the lifespan continuum. Safeedah is in the stage of late adulthood (46–65 years); the practitioner doesn't really appear to have considered her developmental needs in relation to her life stage in the three activities of living.

Your answers in terms of the strengths and limitations could have included the following:

Communication

In this category the practitioner identifies that Safeedah cannot speak English as if it is a problem for her; this is despite the fact that she has not found it an issue in her everyday life before hospitalisation. The practitioner fails to identify her position on the dependence–independence continuum prior to the illness and whether this position has been influenced by her recent diagnosis. The assessment doesn't quantify the extent of her English vocabulary and doesn't mention that she understands the language better than she speaks it. The account omits that she is comfortable talking about her diagnosis and impending treatment. Therefore, in a sense, the assessment doesn't identify what the problem is, whether it is Safeedah or the nurse that has the problem, and how 'big' the problem might be. There is no attempt to assess the coping strategies that Safeedah uses to deal with her lack of independence, such as communicating by simple gestures, or having a close relative who can speak English and is willing to act as an interpreter.

Expressing sexuality

It is not clear from the account how independent Safeedah is in expressing her sexuality. The exploration is limited to a description that really doesn't offer an insight into where Safeedah is on the dependence–independence continuum normally, or how the recent illness and diagnosis may have affected this. The description doesn't really convey any essential information about how Safeedah is coping with the change in dependence. There is no mention of body image or her feelings about her roles and responsibilities related to expressing her sexuality, e.g. mother, wife and homemaker. There are developmental changes that are occurring that will result in physical, sociocultural and psychological needs that are not mentioned in this category. For example, the chances are the treatments ordered by the doctor will affect Safeedah's hormone levels and therefore the process of menstruation or menopause. It is also a time when the success of Safeedah's psychological development rests on feeling that she has a valuable contribution to make to society – a time when she needs to balance supporting her family, friends and wider community by being generous with her knowledge, experience, skills, abilities and time (Erikson 1980). This may prove to be a challenge because of her diagnosis, as there will be a need to divert energies to restoring independence. In turn this may mean a loss of role and/or responsibilities in the family, if only for a short time as she recovers. These are delicate issues and sociocultural factors may have influenced Safeedah's ability to discuss them with the nurse (Baldwin *et al.* 2003). However, to limit the assessment to the brief description offered by the practitioner means that there is a potential to overlook Safeedah's holistic needs.

Dying

It would appear from the assessment that dying was not discussed at all with Safeedah; it is assumed that the practitioner made a professional decision that this activity was too sensitive a topic to explore. However, the activity of dying is much more than the act of dying itself. Think back to Chapter 3 where we explored the category in more detail. The category of dying is concerned with all aspects related to the act of dying – thoughts, fears, concerns, treatments, general beliefs, religious beliefs, rituals, requests and personal wishes. In other words, all the information that would help an individual to carry out this activity in comfort and with respect and dignity. The activity of dying is also about living, and spiritual issues can be explored under this category (McSherry 2007). Safeedah may well have issues related to how she has lived her life, how her life and beliefs and values have changed since her diagnosis, or how her beliefs and values may help her cope with her treatment and experiences. Discussion may need to occur because of the surgery and fears that she may have about her prognosis. It may also be that Safeedah will experience grief as a result of losing her breast, or a role or responsibility that she may have that will be altered as a result of the diagnosis and treatment.

Think about Activity 8.2.

Activity 8.2

Read the scenario of Suzy Clarke in Appendix A. What information gained from your assessment could be included under the activities of communicating, expressing sexuality and dying?

How did you get on with Activity 8.2? Compare your answers with the extracts from Suzy's assessment below.

Communicating

Moved away from home (100 miles) to start nursing programme, 16 months ago. Very close relationship with dad, mum and three sisters, but due to finances only sees them on holiday and phones once a week. Strained relationships with flatmates about sharing of household tasks and house rules. Misses family a lot, arguing/anger seen as way of coping with flatmates and general stressors. Has not contacted the university support services.

Expressing sexuality

Menstruation normally 28 days/5 days moderate to light flow. Uses oral contraception. Now irregular, light flow, 'misses periods' at times, forgets to take contraceptive pill. Usually has good relationship with boyfriend, but now strained; argues all the time. Can see that she sometimes blames boyfriend for her faults and problems. Despite this, boyfriend wants to 'sort things out' and make a go of it.

Dying

States has always been a 'coper', but not coping at the moment – seen GP 10 times in 4 weeks. States 'never been like this, tired, with constant colds and sore throats'. Six weeks ago experienced 'overwhelming sense of impending doom', felt as if she was 'going to suffocate', and thought she 'would die'. **Palpitation**, tightness in chest, sweaty palms, tingling lips and fingers. Admitted to A/E – discharged later that evening – diagnosis 'panic attack'. Has had six further episodes of panic – 'no apparent reason', now very frightened of repeat episodes. Panic rating – 9 at worst and 5 at best, using scale of 1–10. Is very stressed, has high caffeine intake. Convinced there is something seriously wrong – heart problems or brain tumour – that doctors are missing the signs. Full health check given by GP – no abnormalities detected in lungs or heart.

When you look at the three categories it is clear that the practitioner has addressed the first and second stages as identified by RLT and, rather than list the problems, has offered an assessment of Suzy's needs. If you consider the category for dying, the assessment has established the patient's usual routine by offering a description of how Suzy usually carries out the AL; Suzy states that she has always been a 'coper'. It then balances this with a description of her present routine – 'but is not coping at the moment'. This not only offers a judgement as to where Suzy is normally on the dependence–independence continuum in relation to the activity of dying but also highlights whether there has been a change in her level of independence as a consequence of influencing factors. Describing the psychological influencing factor (panic attack) identifies the cause of this movement. The nurse then makes use of subjective and objective information obtained from Suzy herself and offers a brief description of this change in independence: she states that she has 'never been like this, tired, with constant colds and sore throats'. The nurse mentions palpitation, tightness in chest, sweaty palms, tingling lips and fingers and panic rating – 9 at worst and 5 at best, using scale of 1–10.

The assessment then concentrates on describing the adaptive and maladaptive coping strategies that Suzy has adopted as a way of dealing with the problems. Physical coping strategies: palpitation, tightness in chest, sweaty palms, tingling lips and fingers. Psychological coping strategies: is now very frightened of repeat episodes, is convinced that there is something seriously wrong with her and that the doctors are missing the signs of heart problems or a brain tumour.

Finally, there is an account of the nursing care that arises from the interventions/ treatments prescribed or carried out by others: admitted to A/E and discharged later that evening with diagnosis of 'panic attack'. GP has given Suzy a full health check but no abnormalities detected.

Palpitation is the awareness of the beating of your own heart.

Assessment using Orem's Model of Nursing

Orem does not use the word 'assessment', but her term 'nursing history' equates to this stage of the process. The aim of assessing is to:

+ collect information;
+ review and order the information;
+ identify the problems;
+ prioritise the problems.

As we discussed in Chapter 2, a huge number of skills are needed to conduct an assessment. An assessment is not listing problems; it is about establishing the answers to appropriate questions. The assessment could be considered in two stages. In Stage 1 it is important to find out how the patient usually manages their self-care, how they are managing it now and whether there is input from others. The answer to these questions will establish if there is a self-care deficit and how big it is – that is, if there is a change in what the patient could do before and what they can do now in relation to the USCRs. At this point, if there is no deficit identified and the patient is self-caring, then no further questions need to be asked. If a deficit is identified, then you need to investigate further and so you move to Stage 2 of the assessment. Questions 5–8 (listed below) can then be explored. What is causing the change or difference? What they are doing about it? How have they dealt with this in the past (if appropriate)?

A useful tool to help with taking a nursing history is the list of questions that can guide any assessment, whatever the model being used, identified in Chapter 2. We have adapted the questions to use the language that Orem uses and identified a two-stage approach:

Stage 1

1. How self-caring are you normally in the universal self-care requisite (USCR) (or need)? (What can you normally do?)
2. How self-caring are you now in the USCR? (What can you do now?)
3. Is anyone else providing dependent care? (What is anyone else doing about it?)
4. Is there a change or difference in your ability to self-care in the USCRs?
   If no, then no further investigation required.
   If yes, then need to consider the following.

Stage 2

5. Is the change or difference due to a change or lack of knowledge, skill, motivation or behaviour?
6. What is causing the change or difference? Does it derive from a health deviation self-care requisite (HDSCR) (change to structure, function or behaviour) from a developmental self-care requisite (DSCR), or a combination of the two?
7. How are you (with the dependent care agent, if applicable) trying to overcome the self-care deficit? (What are you, or others, doing about it?)
8. How did you deal with this self-care deficit in the past? (How did you deal with the problem in the past?)

As already suggested in Chapter 2, there should be a range of different types of information gathered that includes both objective and subjective information. Orem suggests that, when collecting subjective information, this can include self-statements from the patient. What we mean by this is the use of the patient's own words to describe something; for example, when assessing satisfactory eliminative functions a patient may state that 'It feels like I am passing razor blades when I wee.' The use of the patient's own words emphasises to all concerned the importance of the patient to the whole care-planning process. Using self-statements in the care plan makes ownership by the patient more likely than if it was written using medical jargon, for example 'The patient has pain on micturition.' In Practice example 8.1 there is a small part of an assessment relating to the universal self-care requisite (USCR) of sufficient air intake.

Developmental self-care requisites (DSCRs) should also be considered to see if they have any bearing on the current situation. For example, Albert in Practice example 8.1 has recently been bereaved, which is a significant DSCR. His wife ensured that he took his prescribed antibiotics at the correct time during previous episodes of acute infection; without his wife he has been taking the wrong dose at the wrong times and hence the antibiotics have been ineffective. His wife did all of the food shopping and preparation and, without her, he is not eating a balanced diet; this would be fully explored in the USCR of sufficient intake of water and food. His wife prepaid the gas and he has not taken this commitment over, so the house is not adequately heated; this would be fully explored in the USCR of prevention of hazards to human life, human functioning and human well-being. As you can see, the DSCR of bereavement for Albert is as significant as the health deviation self-care requisite (HDSCR) of acute chest infection and his ability to be self-caring and both need to be explored during the assessment.

Each of the USCRs must be explored to see if there are any deficits in self-care ability. To do this it is essential to find out what the patient could do before and what they can do now; this is the only way you can find out if there is a deficit and how big it is. You may sometimes see problems identified on a care plan without a thorough assessment having taken place; this may lead to problems in the later stages of the process of care planning, for example without knowing the patient's previous routines it would be difficult to set a goal for the patient.

Think about Albert in Practice example 8.1. If the nurse had just concentrated on the acute chest infection (the patient's present ability to self-care) and had not explored his long-standing chronic obstructive pulmonary disease (the patient's previous ability to self-care) then the setting of the goal would be problematic. It is difficult to write a realistic goal if you do not know Albert's previous level of health (returning to self-care). The neighbour was providing dependent care, by helping with the steam inhalations; however, this was not enough to achieve the goal of reducing the therapeutic self-care demand or increasing his capacity to cope with this. Therefore a self-care deficit has been identified that requires nursing intervention and stage 2 of the assessment takes place.

The second stage of the assessment would have established that the self-care deficit is because of a change in structure and function of the lungs due to bacterial infection and his long-standing chronic disorder, a HDSCR. The self-care deficit has been made worse because of a change in behaviour, in the sense that Albert is no longer eating a balanced diet or keeping the house warm, due to his recent bereavement (DSCR). Both of these changes relate to the USCRs of maintaining sufficient intake of water and food and prevention of hazards to health, so these would need to be explored in much more detail. Identifying what is causing the change or difference may be beyond the scope of the patient's ability; the answer may come from laboratory reports, other healthcare professionals or your own clinical knowledge and judgement. However, even following extensive investigation, the cause can remain unknown. This highlights why an experienced nurse needs to be carrying out the assessment, as considerable skill, knowledge, experience and expertise are necessary.

Practice example 8.1

Albert, a 72-year-old man who has recently been bereaved, has been admitted with an acute chest infection; he has existing **chronic obstructive pulmonary disease (COPD)**. Let's use the questions to help to structure the assessment of this USCR.

Stage 1

This stage gives us the opportunity to establish if there is a self-care deficit and how big it is.

1. Usually breathless on exertion, walking over 10 metres. Can usually lie down to sleep. Not usually on oxygen therapy. Non-smoker.

2. Now breathless when at rest. Has to sit in a chair to sleep, as cannot breathe lying down. Here would be included all of the observations about the patient's breathing, colour of skin and mucous membranes, respiratory rate and depth oxygen saturation and oxygen therapy details. Observations of blood pressure and pulse would also be recorded here.

3. Neighbour has been helping with steam inhalations and has been providing food and drinks (food and drink would be fully explored in the USCRs satisfactory intake of water and food).

4. The inhalations helped to start with, but now unable to breathe properly or comfortably; states that 'I can't catch my breath, I feel a bit panicky.'

A deficit exists and so we need to consider questions 5–8.

Stage 2

This stage gives us the opportunity to establish the cause of the deficit and what the patient or dependent-care agent is doing about it.

5. There has been a change in behaviour, in that the patient has not been eating a good diet and has not been heating the house adequately; this has made him more susceptible (more likely) to acquiring infections. (Sometimes there is no obvious change or lack of knowledge, skill, motivation or behaviour.)

6. The change is due to a change in function caused by an acute chest infection (a health deviation self-care deficit), which cannot be overcome, even by a change in behaviour, i.e. sitting up, resting and reducing the demand for oxygen. However, the DSCR of bereavement is also affecting Albert.

7. Went to the doctors and has been taking antibiotics. Trying to reduce the demand for oxygen to the body by keeping still, trying to increase the intake of oxygen by sitting up, well supported by pillows. (The patient may not identify their attempts to reduce their demand for oxygen and how they are trying to increase the intake, but they would tell you what they are doing.)

8. In the past when Albert had an acute infection, he used steam inhalations and went to the doctors for antibiotics. His wife ensured that he took his medication as prescribed, which he is no longer doing.

Chronic obstructive pulmonary disease (COPD) is a progressive and long-standing disease of the lungs.

Finding out what the patient is doing, or has done in the past, to overcome the self-care deficit gives us an idea of the types of behaviour the patient will engage in to promote self-care. We also need to find out whether the strategies they are using are making the healthcare deficit better (adaptive coping strategies) or making the deficit worse (maladaptive coping strategies), as discussed in the chapter on ASPIRE. Orem's philosophy is to promote self-care, and therefore it is crucial to find out how the patient is coping with the change in self-care. If the coping strategy is a productive or adaptive one that helps meet the problem, then it needs to be encouraged and extended. If it is not helping the problem or it is a maladaptive coping strategy, then it should be discouraged and other more positive behaviours encouraged. This will influence the stage of the nursing process concerned with giving the care (implementation), as wherever possible nursing actions should be organised around the patient's current ways of dealing with the universal self-care requisites and seek to build upon these routines. As we've already discussed, this is because it is often easier to modify an existing behaviour than try to introduce a brand new one. Additionally, patients are more likely to consent to and comply with a plan of care if it is founded upon their existing ways of coping.

Consideration of the input of others – family, friends, carers (those providing dependent care) or other healthcare providers – is relevant to the assessment. The overriding message of Orem's philosophy is to promote self-care (independence). This means that you need to be careful not to step in and perform any activities for the patient unless you really have to; therefore, it makes sense to identify the input of friends and family as their actions may be ensuring that the universal self-care requisites are met and nursing input may not be required.

Once you have conducted the assessment process you will need to categorise the information under the appropriate USCR. As with the activities of living, this doesn't mean that we should use the USCRs as a checklist. Instead, they are a prompt to help us remember the complexity of an individual's life. The conversations between you and your patients should be as natural as possible, letting them disclose their experiences of carrying out self-care in each USCR so that you can identify the problems together.

A full detailed account of the assessment is necessary to allow everyone access to an accurate picture of the patient's needs (present and near future) and how they are affecting their ability to carry out self-care in each USCR. The assessment should offer a description of how self-caring the patient is; this information should in turn be set against the 'normal routine' for that patient.

The information gathered and categorised under the headings should facilitate the discovery of actual and potential problems, the identification of need statements and baselines, the setting of the goals and the establishing of available resources to meet these goals. A thorough assessment is one that provides information to make the next stages of care planning much easier to carry out. The problem is that, if the assessment process is not adhered to or is not as thorough as it should be, then the next stages will be difficult and reflect the shortfalls of the procedure. This means a thorough assessment is one that includes all of the necessary information that makes the next stages comprehensive and should provide the means to give safe and effective care to the patient, which is the ultimate goal of planning care.

The information gathered when taking a nursing history (assessment) needs to be adequately documented following the guidelines of record keeping as prescribed by the NMC (2009a). For this to happen there needs to be a well-designed format, whether that be handwritten or computerised (as discussed in Chapter 7), to ensure all of the information is available to the patient and the nursing team that will be caring for the patient. Nurses may find that there is limited space to document all of the information found at assessment; this means that much of it is lost from the care-planning process. The forms should be tailored to the information required, rather than the information being tailored to the forms.

Now look at Activity 8.3.

Activity 8.3

Consider the following examples of part of a nursing history taken by a nurse using Orem's model.

1. Balance between solitude and social interactions − no problems.
2. Promotion of human functioning and development within social groups in accordance with human potential, known human limitations and the desire for normalcy − likes to wear make-up.
3. Prevention of hazards to human life, functioning and well-being − loose rug, house electrics require maintenance.

What do you think of these examples? Think about what you would like to see in each one if you were going to nurse the patient.

How did you do with Activity 8.3? The information categorised under number 1 is not an example of a nursing history; it does not answer any of the questions that are used to guide an assessment. The answers to all of the questions from stage 1 should be included. How self-caring are you normally in the USCR? How self-caring are you now in the USCR? Is anyone else providing dependent care? Is there a change or difference in your ability to self-care in the USCRs? If there is no change or difference, then there is no need to go to stage 2, but the answers to the first questions need to be recorded in the nursing history. This is because it is as important to know what USCRs the patients can carry out for themselves as it is to establish those that have a self-care deficit. In addition, as the USCRs are interdependent, information recorded under one category may prove useful when carrying out the rest of the nursing history and the other stages of the care-planning process.

The information in example 2 in Activity 8.3 would be included in the nursing history of this USCR, as it gives some indication of the patient's self-concept, but far more information would be required to explore this USCR fully. It is important to remember that this USCR represents a person's ability to regulate themselves physically, psychologically and socially. It also refers to the individual's drive to maintain and promote their structure and function and their own development. Information relating to a patient's role concept would need to be included; for example do they see themselves primarily as a wife and mother, or as a breadwinner, or both?

When considering the third example the nurse has concentrated on identifying hazards in the external environment; whilst these are relevant, there would also be a need to consider information about hazards within the internal environment, as discussed previously. Once again, the nurse has not conducted a nursing history, but merely listed problems or hazards.

Look at Activity 8.4.

Activity 8.4

Read the scenario of George Brown in Appendix B. What information would you identify from taking a nursing history for the USCRs for sufficient intake of air and the balance between solitude and social interaction?

Compare your nursing history from Activity 8.4 with the following accounts taken from George's care plan in Appendix B.

Sufficient intake of air

George did smoke 20 years ago (20 per day for 40 years) and, although he has a chronic non-productive cough, he has no breathing or circulatory problems. He has a pale/sallow complexion but his mucous membranes are pink. No history of anaemia, blood test results are within normal limits, haemoglobin 11.8 grams/100 millilitres (12.11.12). Respirations 14 per minute, B/P 140/90, pulse 90 beats per minute, good volume, rhythmic.

George's assessment relating to sufficient intake of air answers all of the questions in stage 1; because a deficit has not been identified, there is no need to progress to stage 2. However, this decision cannot be made until you have completed the first stage. You will note that there is sufficient information here to deduce that there are no problems, not simply a statement of 'no problems'. Other care workers looking after George who did not take the nursing history can see the relevant information about this USCR and, if problems arise in the future relating to this, they have a baseline to work with.

Balance between solitude and social interaction

Retired to the seaside town four years ago, after very much looking forward to retirement from his job as head gardener to the parks department very much. He has one son and two grandsons who live in a city about 13 miles away. George and his wife Elsie say they are very close to their family, and used to lead a busy social life, meeting with friends 3–4 times a week for coffee, lunch or an evening meal at the local pub. Now they are not going out with their friends at all. George usually uses hearing aid to achieve good levels of communication and can lip-read very well. Is profoundly deaf and has become reluctant to use his hearing aid (past three months); he is finding he doesn't want to mix with his friends and doesn't look forward to his family visiting. Elsie says 'I really miss seeing our friends but I don't feel I can leave George on his own.' George says he is fed-up and 'tired', often choosing to turn off his hearing aid when friends and family visit. Elsie manages the home and the finances (she always has done). George relies upon her support, guidance and judgement greatly.

George's nursing history relating to solitude and social interaction has more informa-tion due to a deficit being identified; therefore you need the answers to both the first and second stages of the process, rather than list problems. The assessment has established the patient's usual routine by offering a description of how George usually carries out the USCR: Usually uses hearing aid to achieve good levels of communication and can lip-read very well. It then balances this with a description of his present routine – George says he is fed-up and tired, often choosing to turn off his hearing aid when friends and family visit. This not only offers a judgement as to how George normally is with regard to being self-caring in relation to the USCR of balance between solitude and social interaction but also highlights whether there has been a change in his level of independence as a consequence of other factors. Describing the change in behaviour – feeling fed-up and tired – identifies the cause of this movement. The nurse then makes use of subjective and objective information obtained from George and Elsie. There is a record of the number and types of social interactions that occurred, previously and now.

Note that there are a number of self-statements from George and Elsie; this means that they can be used when writing the care plan. Using self-statements means that George and Elsie are more likely to have ownership of the plan, places George at the centre of the proc-ess and helps them understand the terms used.

Assessment using the Neuman Systems Model

To look at how the the Neuman Systems Model (NSM) can help with assessment, you'll need to refer to the Shoaib Hameed scenario in Appendix C. We're going to think about how Shoaib could be assessed following transfer to the ward from the coronary care unit. Bear in mind that the acute phase of Shoaib's care is now complete, and that he is now at the start of a process of recovery and rehabilitation.

You should also remember the fundamentals of assessment that apply *whatever* nursing model is being used. We've already touched on these within this chapter, but they are so impor-tant that it doesn't hurt to have another look – you'll find a list of key points in Exhibit 8.1.

> + You should aim to find out how the patient was before they developed problems, and how they are now.
> + You should always try to identify coping strategies, whether adaptive or maladaptive.
> + You should always try to discover why a particular problem has occurred: it is not enough simply to document that a problem exists.

Exhibit 8.1 Key points for assessment

In her model, Betty Neuman provides a step-by-step tool for carrying out assessment and intervention. Many clinical areas will adapt this to meet their own needs, but we'll look at it as prescribed by Neuman herself. Before working through the assessment of Shoaib, it is worth familiarising yourself again with the principles of Neuman's model in Chapter 5.

We'll look at the ins and outs of using the model in a moment, but it is just worth high-lighting the three principles that will run through any NSM-based assessment. First, any assessment should give you knowledge of all the factors influencing a patient's perception of the world. This idea bears some resemblance to the exploration of influencing factors appar-ent in the Activities of Living Model. Secondly, an assessment should be focused around the patient and the effect that different stressors are having on them – any findings should there-fore be agreed by the patient and the nurse carrying out the assessment. Finally, Neuman talks in some detail about the need for you as a carer to be aware of reasons that may influence your perception of the patient (for example, past experiences or personal biases).

As with all models, assessment with the NSM starts with the gathering of biographical data and information regarding referral. You would therefore use all the available sources of information – e.g. Shoaib himself, the medical notes – to gain a clear picture of his background and medical history to date. After this point, assessment with Neuman's model becomes rather different from that with the Activities of Living or Self-Care models. Rather than breaking down the patient into different activities or elements, we simply need to think about the stressors that are influencing the patient. First of all, we ask for the patient's perception of their stressors. Neuman provides us with six questions that can be asked of the patient about the stressors:

1. What are your major stress areas or health concerns?
2. How are these circumstances different from normal?
3. Have you had similar problems before? How did you handle this?
4. How do you view the future as a consequence of this situation?
5. What are you doing (and what can you do) to help yourself?
6. What do you expect others to do for you?

As with all nursing models, you need to use a bit of common sense when putting it into practice. If you used the exact terminology prescribed by Neuman when asking questions, the patient (and your colleagues) might look at you in a rather strange way. To try to simplify things, it might be easier to think of the general point of the questions asked within the NSM assessment:

1. What's worrying you?
2. How are things different from normal?
3. Have you had this before? What did you do about it?
4. How do you think this is going to affect your future?
5. What are you doing to help yourself?
6. What do you want us (the nurses), your family and friends to do?

Even these simplified questions may not be appropriate for everyone, but they are a useful starting point.

STOP AND THINK

Why do you think it is so useful to ask the patient questions about their perceptions of their health problems and the impact that these are likely to have on their future?

The reason behind the list of questions is simple: it allows you to get an idea of what the patient is worrying about, but it also highlights any misconceptions that they may have. Thinking about Shoaib for a moment, let's consider the thing that is worrying him the most, which, understandably, is the fact that he has suffered a myocardial infarction (or a 'heart attack' in layperson terms). By asking Shoaib about his perceptions of the future and the care that he needs, you'll get a really good idea of his level of knowledge and how realistic his outlook is. He may, for example, think that the heart attack will mean that he must give up work and will be housebound for years to come – something that is unlikely to be the case and can be clarified early on. It's also important to realise that these six questions are just part of a framework for assessment, and you'll also need to ask some more specific questions to get more detail.

Once you've asked Shoaib the six questions, then the next step is to ask them again, but this time of yourself. In other words:

1. What are the patient's major stress areas or health concerns?
2. How are these circumstances different from normal?
3. Has the patient had similar problems before? How did he handle this?
4. How do you view the future as a consequence of this situation?
5. What is the patient doing (and what can he do) to help himself?
6. What should others be expected to do to help the patient?

Asking these questions of yourself allows you to get an idea of what is worrying you about the patient's well-being. Try Activity 8.5 to have a run-through of using the six-question approach.

Activity 8.5

Read through Shoaib's scenario in Appendix C. Think about three areas of health concern that you might have for a patient such as Shoaib, and try to answer the six questions for each of them. It doesn't matter if you don't know much about cardiac care; just take a guess at the problems and implications.

How did you get on with Activity 8.5? You may have thought of a number of health concerns that Shoaib has, and tried to think through the possible answers. For example, the most obvious health concern is that Shoaib has had a myocardial infarction (MI), so that's one answer for question 1. Shoaib has never had an MI before, so this is completely different from normal (question 2), and he has never had a similar problem (question 3). Question 4 is where your expertise really comes to the fore. After an MI, concerns about the future include the possibility of complications (such as the heart starting to fail), the chance of another MI months or years in the future, and the possibility of the patient not returning to their previous state of health. Question 5 would ask about Shoaib's own input into his care at the moment, and question 6 would allow you to assess the care being provided by the healthcare team to aid Shoaib's recovery.

After completing this stage of the assessment, you've got a lot of information about the patient. You know what is concerning them, and have ascertained what their perceptions and knowledge are about these problems. You've also had the opportunity to reflect on what you are concerned about with regard to your patient, and think about the care that is currently being delivered.

The next step is to summarise of the patient's condition as viewed by you and the patient, taking care to note any differences between the patient's views and yours. The fact that you will come across situations in which you and the patient have different views on the stressors is not a problem. As we've already highlighted, this helps you identify where the patient (or you) has distorted views on a particular issue, and allows an opportunity to 'iron out' these misconceptions.

Neuman provides a clear structure for summarising the assessment findings. Broadly speaking, the summary is split into three headings that we've already discussed within Chapter 5: intrapersonal, interpersonal and extrapersonal.

If you remember from Chapter 5, intrapersonal factors relate to those things that happen within us. In relation to assessment, these intrapersonal factors are split further into physical, psychosociocultural, developmental and spiritual headings. In Shoaib's case, a physical factor might be the fact that he has suffered an MI; a pyschosociocultural factor might be his very strong work ethic and tendency to do too much; a developmental factor might be his particular age and his initial wish to retire; a spiritual factor could be the support offered by his faith. Table 8.1 demonstrates our complete summary of Shoaib's assessment.

Table 8.1 Shoaib Hameed assessment summary

Intrapersonal

Physical

Myocardial infarction 48 hours ago
Has been commenced on aspirin, dopidogrel, beta-blocker, ACE inhibitor and statin
Currently pain-free – taking no analgesia
Bruising in right groin following PCI
O_2 saturation now 99% on air (norm is 95–100%)
BP 110/60mmHg, pulse rate 75 bpm
Smokes 30 cigarettes per day
Has attempted to give up smoking 3 times in the past 12 months with no nicotine replacement therapy
Weight 101.6kg (16 stone), height 1.8m (5'11') (BMI 32)
Doesn't drink alcohol due to religious beliefs
Has a balanced diet at home. However, diet at work is poor – usually skips lunch. Has high-fat diet when away on business
Total cholesterol 6.4mmol, LDL cholesterol 4.3mmol, HDL cholesterol 1mmol
Has not opened bowels since admission – feels constipated and is scared of straining in case he gets more chest pain
Normally opens bowels every day
Eating small amounts, but does not like hospital food
Is wary about mobilising to the toilet due to fear of getting more chest pain, so using urine bottles most of the time
Is managing to wash most of himself with a bowl at his bed. Needs help with washing his back
Is only wearing pyjamas at present – able to dress independently
Would like to shower but is scared of suffering another MI whilst in bathroom
Has been reluctant to exercise recently due to experiencing shoulder pain on exertion
Is mobilising very gently, but is concerned about doing too much in case pain returns
Normally sleeps 4 hours per night – goes to bed late and wakes at about 5.30 a.m., worrying about work
Sleeping poorly (<2 hours per night) due to noise on CCU and anxiety about condition
Reluctant to have sleeping pills in case he gets addicted

Psychosociocultural

Smokes because he feels stressed about work and money
No hearing or speech problems. Wears glasses for driving and watching TV
Stressful job – manager in IT firm. Works 14 hours a day and takes work home
Comfortable lifestyle but little time to enjoy it
Large house and mortgage
Strong work ethic
Is unhappy with size and fitness – feels that he has 'let himself go'

Developmental

Is keen to do whatever is necessary to recover from his MI and prevent further events
Had originally planned to retire to south of France at 55 but commitments have changed these plans

Spiritual

Very anxious, scared that he is going to die
Muslim faith
Feels that his Muslim faith will help him through this experience

Interpersonal

Jokes with family about being overweight
Quite withdrawn and quiet. Little interaction with healthcare team or other patients
Feels that he has little to talk about with other patients
Often feels isolated at work, and does not get enough opportunity to mix with family and friends
Has good relationship with wife and children, although it is strained by his long hours of work
Wife and children visit regularly and want to get involved in care
Shoaib feels isolated at times in hospital – 'nothing in common with other patients'
Close bond with wife
Believes that sexual relations with his wife may not be possible due to MI

Extrapersonal

Is worried about financial implications of illness
Is worried about the effects of his illness on his work colleagues

Let's take stock of where we are at the moment. After the four stages of assessing a patient using Neuman's model you will have got all the biographical and clinical details that you need. You'll also have insight into the patient's views on their condition and problems, and have had the opportunity to explore your main concerns. Finally, you will have a structured summary of what has been found during the assessment – just like the one in Table 8.1. This summary provides the starting point for the next stage of care planning: systematic nursing diagnosis. We'll look at how to develop a nursing diagnosis for Shoaib in the next chapter, but for now it is just useful to reflect on the assessment process within the Neuman Systems Model.

Neuman's view of assessment is much 'looser' than that described by Roper, Logan and Tierney or by Orem. There is no prescribed list of activities or requisites to assess, which does remove the risk of assessment becoming a checklist. The more open approach to assessment also recognises the importance of gaining the patient's viewpoint on their condition, and allows nurses to use their clinical expertise in highlighting what they believe the factors affecting the patient are.

On the downside, the lack of structure may be difficult if you are less experienced and confident in the assessment of patients. If this is the case, then there is no reason why nursing models can't be used together to give the best result. You could use the structure of the Activities of Living or Self-Care Requisites to help structure the assessment, whilst using the approach of Neuman's model (asking the six key questions of the patient, and then asking yourself the same) to assess each of these elements. The key is to use models in such a way that they help you as much as possible.

Conclusion

Within this chapter, we've looked at assessment using three nursing models. Some elements of assessment are the same, whichever model you use. For example, you will always need to gather baseline biographical and health information, ascertain normal and current health status, consider the role played by friends and family and consider the patient's own views on their condition.

In other areas, the assessment stage might be very different depending on the model used. RLT and Orem tend to have a slightly more structured set of prompts for assessment (the ALs and USCRs). This does increase the danger of 'checklist' assessment if you don't use the model properly, but it does make assessment easier for a less experienced nurse. Neuman's assessment process is much looser: this makes it a little more dependent on your own clinical judgement to make it work, but it is less restrictive than other models.

Whichever model you use, the assessment stage is crucial as a starting point of care planning. Through a comprehensive assessment, you will gain the information that you need to move on to the next stage – systematic nursing diagnosis.

Chapter 9

Systematic nursing diagnosis

Why this chapter matters

Nursing diagnosis differs from medical diagnosis, because nursing diagnosis focuses on the consequences of living with a set of signs and symptoms or the medical diagnosis. Let's think about a really simple example: a patient goes to their GP complaining of problems with opening their bowels. The GP, after carrying out an assessment, diagnoses constipation and prescribes medication. If a practice nurse sees the patient, then the systematic nursing diagnosis may focus more on the consequences of living with constipation: the patient feels bloated, dizzy or nauseous, or they do not understand what constipation is or what causes it. It then follows that the interventions leading from this process of systematic nursing diagnosis will be different to that prescribed by the GP. Also, the care will place greater emphasis on making the patient comfortable, reassuring them and offering them advice about diet and exercise. The nursing intervention would also involve making sure that the patient understands the medication, how to take it and what side effects to look for. Although nurses offer care that is complementary to that prescribed by the GP, we also offer a unique contribution that is identifiable as nursing care.

In this chapter we will concentrate on the second stage of the ASPIRE approach – systematic nursing diagnosis – and offer explorations of how this stage may be carried out using Roper, Logan and Tierney's Activities of Living Model, Orem's Self-Care Model of Nursing and the Neuman Systems Model.

By the end of the chapter you will be able to:

+ list the steps that lead to systematic nursing diagnosis;

+ conduct a systematic nursing diagnosis using Roper, Logan and Tierney's Activities of Living Model, Orem's Self-Care Model of Nursing and the Neuman Systems Model.

Systematic nursing diagnosis using the Activities of Living Model

In this stage, the patient's nursing needs are identified from the assessment, along with the appropriate baselines. Remember that a baseline offers a description or measurement of 'where the patient is now' in relation to the need. It provides information that will prove crucial in judging the patient's progress towards the identified goal during the ongoing and final evaluation stage. Once the nursing diagnosis is made, a clear need statement and baseline are agreed with the patient. When you write the need statement it is important to consider the philosophy that underpins the Roper, Logan and Tierney (RLT) model. With this in mind, you can use the five key concepts/ideas from the model to help you:

+ individuality;
+ the activities of living;
+ the dependence–independence continuum;
+ the progression of a person along a lifespan continuum;
+ influencing factors.

Finally, the needs are prioritised, a process that should be patient-led, though you may have to seek advice from the relatives/friends if the patient is unable to act or do for themselves (Dimond, 2011).

Consider Activity 9.1.

Activity 9.1

Helen is an 18-year-old student admitted to the ward as an emergency admission after collapsing and falling into unconsciousness at home. The doctor diagnoses **type 1 diabetes mellitus** and the condition is stabilised over a 36-hour period. Helen is working towards a discharge date but confides that she is very worried about her future. She is due to go to university in a few months and is very concerned about coping with the diabetes, especially because she has a needle phobia and doesn't understand the condition at all. Helen has heard that diabetes 'makes you fat' so is worried about gaining weight and she is also fearful that she won't be able to do the things that she likes to do, such as clubbing with her friends and going to the gym.

The nurse makes a diagnosis and writes the need statement in Helen's care plan; she is using RLT as the model of choice to underpin the stages of ASPIRE. The need statement produced for Helen is: 'Helen has diabetes mellitus'.

Can you identify the strengths and limitations of the need statement?

Type I diabetes mellitus is a disease resulting from no natural production of insulin, a hormone that helps control blood glucose levels.

How did you get on with Activity 9.1? Perhaps the biggest concern with this need statement is that it is not based upon a nursing diagnosis. It is a medical diagnosis that emphasises changes and needs that are physical or biological in nature, e.g. lack of insulin and control of blood glucose levels with diet and medication. This reflects a reductionist approach, one that reduces the information to one possible cause. A nursing diagnosis places emphasis on the holistic needs of the patient by considering the physical, psychological, social and spiritual consequences that arise from owning a particular set of signs and symptoms or medical diagnosis. Helen's need statement – 'Helen has diabetes mellitus' – is really a medical label, and as such fails to identify what Helen's nursing needs are. This makes the need statement unclear and ambiguous for any nurse trying to deliver Helen's care, because it is too vague and imprecise. It is also unlikely that Helen has any ownership of the problem, especially as the statement doesn't identify her nursing needs and uses language that could be seen as exclusive. This may increase the likelihood of Helen not following or contributing to her plan of care. Lastly, the attempt at the need statement doesn't really emphasise or make use of the key five elements as suggested by RLT; it fails to reflect the philosophy of RLT and as such is not personal to Helen.

Let's explore the issues in a little more depth. RLT propose that nursing intervention is more than treating the medical label: it is holistic in its approach, and therefore it is not just the illness/disease that requires nursing care but the person. The systematic nursing diagnosis should have identified the needs that arise from living with diabetes. It needs to concentrate on the consequences the signs and symptoms or medical diagnosis have on Helen's life – how she will cope with going to the gym or clubbing with her friends, leaving home to go to university or dealing with her needle phobia. Think about the issues that were raised in Chapter 1 and the legal, ethical and professional implications of not identifying or carrying out care. It is easy to see how problems are overlooked as a consequence of focusing on the medical diagnosis rather than the nursing diagnosis. That is not to say you do not have to deal with the physical problems that accompany a medical diagnosis, but there will be needs that arise from psychological, social and spiritual aspects related to that illness or disease that need to be identified and addressed.

The nurse in activity 9.1 was meant to be using RLT's Activities of Living Model and therefore the philosophy should have influenced the systematic nursing diagnosis and underpinned the need statement. Yet the five key points of individuality, dependence–independence continuum (what they cannot or can do), activities of living, the influencing factors (what is causing the problem) and the lifespan continuum are not evident in the statement.

Finally, there are no baselines to personalise the care and identify where Helen is now in relation to the need. This means that goal setting would be more difficult because there isn't a record of where she is now to help establish where she would like to be in the near future. One of the baselines informs you that she cannot draw up the insulin and inject herself because of her needle phobia, so a goal could be set in agreement with Helen that she will be able to draw up her insulin and inject herself by an agreed date. The baselines would also help you identify the prescription of care to deal with the problem, e.g. address the needle phobia and lack of knowledge about the condition. Baselines help you to individualise the care and include all of the problems that arise from living with the signs and symptoms or medical diagnosis. One last thing to highlight is that goals are the criteria we use to evaluate whether the prescribed care has been successful or not; but without baselines you cannot really make an informed decision as to whether there has been movement away or towards the goal. Identifying the baseline in the assessment allows you to make a judgement as to the degree of Helen's progress.

Helen's situation calls for more than one need statement to deal with her problems of living with diabetes, However, one example that endorses the philosophy of the activities of Living model could be;

Helen says she is worried about maintaining her lifestyle due to her lack of knowledge about diabetes mellitus:

Baselines:

+ worry score 3 at best and 9 at worst on a scale of 0-10
+ no knowledge about diabetes and management
+ Helen has read that diabetes makes you fat – current weight is 57 kg (8st 11lb)
+ Helen feels that she no longer has any control over her life – cannot go to university in Sept, go clubbing, go to the gym
+ 'control score' 2 at best and 10 at worst on a scale of 0-10

Managing her blood glucose levels, diet and exercise and addressing her fear of needles would call for additional need statements and baselines. However, can you see how a nursing diagnosis adopts a holistic approach to care planning when compared to the reductionist approach that underpinned the medical diagnosis of 'Helen has diabetes mellitus'? This biopsychosocial approach is only possible if a comprehensive, holistic assessment has been conducted.

Activity 9.2

Consider the scenario for Suzy Clarke and her diagnosis of thrush (Appendix A). Write a need statement that reflects the five key concepts of the RLT model. Don't forget to include a baseline (a description of where the patient is now).

How did you do with Activity 9.2? It should look something like this: Suzy says she has pain when 'passing urine', due to thrush.

Baselines:

+ pain is 6 on scale of 1–10; 'burns and stings' when passing urine, feels miserable
+ vaginal redness, white discharge, yeasty odour
+ itching at worst 8 and at best 5 on comfort scale of 1–10
+ high vaginal swab – results on 17.10.12 positive to *Candida albicans*

What this example offers is a clear unambiguous statement that is individualised because it relates to Suzy and the consequences that arise from living with her medical diagnosis. Because we are using the Activities of Living Model, it offers a nursing diagnosis that describes how the thrush is affecting her ability to carry out the activities of living. The need statement identifies the activity of living that she cannot do (eliminating – pass urine) and confirms that there has been movement along the dependence–independence continuum (what she can and cannot do) caused by a physical influencing factor (the infection). There are descriptions of baselines that represent where Suzy is now in relation to the problem;

this introduces an individual, personal element to the care and will prove invaluable when setting the goals, deciding the prescription of care and evaluating the outcome later in the ASPIRE process. What this does show is how each of the ASPIRE stages are dependent on one another.

We have explored the difference between medical diagnosis and nursing diagnosis and how to write a need statement and baseline using the Activities of Living Model. However, we almost need to go back a step and reconsider what systematic nursing diagnosis entails to try to demonstrate how nurses establish the problems from the assessment and come up with a systematic nursing diagnosis.

When offering a medical diagnosis a doctor will often consider all the possible problems that arise from the signs and symptoms and offer a single diagnosis; by reducing all the possibilities to the one thing that is causing the effect, usually a biological cause. This is a reductionist approach. Nursing diagnosis is about establishing the problems that a patient has as a consequence of living with the signs or symptoms and the medical diagnosis. This means that we have to start with the signs and symptoms or medical diagnosis and establish the nursing problems that originate from this label. This is a holistic approach.

The list is usually large in number; this is because nursing care is about dealing with a patient's holistic needs and, as discussed, these are often interrelated and interdependent making it even more confusing. However, there is a need to diagnose the nursing problem without missing anything that may interfere with the patient's recovery. Therefore, at some point, you need to make a decision as to what the main issues are and how the other issues relate and are dependent on them, in order to come up with a nursing diagnosis: this is what we refer to as systematic nursing diagnosis.

Remember in Chapter 2 we said that it is often possible for nurses to develop diagnoses extremely quickly and without apparent effort because of their knowledge and expertise. However, even when it is not apparent, the systematic approach first discussed in Chapter 2 is still being used:

+ An assessment takes place using theoretical knowledge and past expertise
+ Analysis takes place and possible problems are identified
+ Critical thinking allows identification of how the problems are interrelated and interdependent
+ Critical analysis allows a conclusion to be made by establishing the nursing diagnosis; this is based on the consequences of living with the signs and symptoms or medical diagnosis
+ Synthesis allows you to write a need statement and baselines to reflect this nursing diagnosis
+ The nursing diagnosis is confirmed by going back to the patient to clarify that the problems have been included in the need statement and that it represents their experience.

Systematic nursing diagnosis requires the use of knowledge and skills that develop over time and needs lots of practice. To help, we'll use this chapter to give some examples of how that six-stage process of nursing diagnosis can result in useful, patient-focused need statements.

An assessment takes place using theoretical knowledge and past expertise. Using the first and second stage of assessing, a holistic and comprehensive assessment is conducted as described in Chapter 8. An example of this can be found in Suzy's care plan (see appendix A).

Analysis takes place and possible problems are identified. Analysis is where you break information down into smaller parts. In other words, you identify the important points or main features so that you can examine these in close detail. In the case of care planning you analyse by identifying and listing the actual and potential problems from the assessment. When using RLT's model the problems are established by identifying a change in the patient's present routine when compared to their previous routines, in relation to one or more of the activities of living; this change reflects movement along the dependence–independence continuum as a result of one or more of the influencing factors.

A list of Suzy's problems could look like this:

+ damp, cold house, outstanding repairs;
+ unhelpful landlord;
+ overdrawn at the bank;
+ anaemic (iron deficiency); low Hb and ferritin levels
+ frequent headaches;
+ moved away from home to start nursing programme;
+ misses family contacts and sees them only occasionally;
+ feels unsafe and lonely;
+ strained relationship with flatmates and landlord;
+ argues with boyfriend;
+ smokes;
+ non-productive cough;
+ alcohol intake has increased;
+ diet high in fat, carbohydrates, sugars; low in protein, fresh fruit and vegetables;
+ sore, red throat;
+ drinks large amounts of cola;
+ cuts back on heating and food costs;
+ weight loss;
+ constipated;
+ thrush – vaginal redness, itching and white discharge;
+ unaware of the trigger factors for thrush;
+ has unprotected sex with boyfriend;
+ breathless on exertion;
+ reduced sleep pattern;
+ naps through the day;
+ fallen behind with university work;
+ panic attacks;
+ thinks that she has something seriously wrong with her;
+ thinks the GP is missing signs and symptoms;

+ dizzy on standing;
+ frequent headaches;
+ feels exhausted;
+ night sweats.

Critical thinking allows identification of how the problems are interrelated and interdependent. Obviously, we can't plan care for all of these problems individually, but we don't really need to. Much of your nursing practice (and academic activity) requires you to carry out critical thinking. This calls for the ability to be able to compare and contrast information. The key to diagnosing nursing problems in a systematic way is to use this skill of comparing and contrasting to establish how problems relate to each other and are dependent on each other. For example, Suzy has a problem of anaemia, but looking down the list, using your skills of critical thinking allows you to see that the problems of headaches, breathlessness on exertion, dizziness on standing and feeling exhausted are all related to the problem of anaemia and each other. It would make sense then to group these problems together – this is an example of how problems are *interrelated*. However, the reduced sleep pattern and night sweats are dependent on the anaemia in the sense that if the anaemia is addressed, the sleep pattern will improve and the night sweats will be alleviated or eliminated over time – this is an example of problems that are *interdependent*. Equally, the signs and symptoms of panic attack need to be grouped together because they are interrelated (see Table 9.1), but if we prescribe interventions to help Suzy become independent in dealing with her panic attacks, she will not think that there is something seriously wrong with her or that the GP is failing her by overlooking or missing signs and symptoms. This false perception of believing she is seriously ill is dependent on the panic attacks; if we deal with the panic attacks the misperception of her illness will be alleviated and eliminated over time.

It is plain to see that systematic nursing diagnosis is a skill that takes knowledge and time to develop. A knowledgeable, experienced nurse would be able to make the decision as to which problems are interrelated and which ones are interdependent, so that she can make sense of the problems by collapsing them or grouping them together. Consider the grouping of Suzy's problems in terms of how they are interrelated and interdependent (see Table 9.1).

An added dimension to the grouping of Suzy's problems is that because we are using RLT's model we can categorise the groups of problems under the appropriate activity of living to establish exactly how the problems are affecting her. For example, the group of interrelated and interdependent problems 'feels exhausted, frequent headaches, anaemia, breathless on exertion dizzy on standing, reduced sleep patterns and night sweats' are categorised under the AL of 'mobility'. This is because Suzy is highlighting how these are affecting her ability to be as active as she previously was. It is not necessary to include a problem under every one of the activities of living, and it is also perfectly acceptable to have more than one problem under one of the headings, as we have done with Suzy in the case of 'maintaining a safe environment'. The placing of the problems in the appropriate category of 12 activities of living is meant to help you focus your attention towards the activity of living it is affecting and to create some order from the chaos of the large list of problems. This task will also help you to write your need statement because you will have already considered which of the activities Suzy is having problems carrying out.

Table 9.1 Systematic nursing diagnosis for Suzy Clarke

Maintaining a safe environment	
Panic attacks	● Overwhelming sense of 'impending doom' ● Palpitation, tightness in chest, sweaty palms, tingling lips and fingers during panic episodes ● Thinks that she has something seriously wrong with her ● Thinks the GP is overlooking or missing the signs and symptoms
Not coping – feels unsafe and lonely	● Overdrawn at the bank ● Cuts back on heating and food costs ● Fallen behind with university work, not coping with demands of nursing programme ● Strained relationship with flatmates ● Argues with boyfriend and flatmates ● Smokes ● Non-productive cough ● Reduced sleep pattern ● Naps through the day
Eating and drinking/eliminating	
Not eating well-balanced diet	● Drinks large amounts of cola ● Constipated ● Loss of weight ● Anaemic ● Sore, red throat
Eliminating/expressing sexuality	
Pain on passing urine	● Thrush ● Vaginal redness, itching and white discharge ● Unaware of trigger factors for thrush ● Unprotected sex with boyfriend
Mobility	
Feels exhausted	● Frequent headaches ● Anaemic – low hb and ferritin levels ● Breathless on exertion ● Dizzy on standing ● Reduced pattern of sleep ● Night sweats

Critical analysis allows a conclusion to be made by establishing the nursing diagnosis; this is based on the consequences of living with the signs and symptoms or medical diagnosis. In the past, you may have had to complete pieces of academic work that call for the demonstration of critical analysis. To do this, you have to sum up your discussions in one clear, brief sentence that states your position, then convince the reader of your decision by persuading them that the evidence leads to the conclusion that you have arrived at. You also need to use these skills of critical analysis when you make a nursing diagnosis; this means you focus on the group of problems and identify with the patient how the signs and symptoms or medical diagnosis is affecting them. In other words, you identify what the consequences of living with these problems are. If you have conducted a comprehensive, holistic assessment, the groups of problems should reflect the biopsychosocial needs of the patient and allow you to make a nursing diagnosis that is individual to that patient. Whilst you do not necessarily have to convince someone else that the evidence leads to the conclusion that you have arrived at in the way that you do when writing an essay, you will be expected to be able to offer a rationale for your diagnosis and be prepared to demonstrate how you arrived at your conclusion.

Synthesis allows you to write a need statement and baselines to reflect this nursing diagnosis. The skills of synthesis require you to recombine various points from your thought processes to help develop a new idea or suggestion – in this case, a need statement that reflects the nursing diagnosis. Consider the list of problems under Mobility in Table 9.1, and the need statement: 'Suzy says she is "exhausted", has frequent headaches and feels dizzy when standing from a sitting position due to anaemia.'

This need statement reflects the nursing diagnosis for Suzy (that is, what it is like to live with the problems in the list). Because we are using the Activities of Living Model, it offers a nursing diagnosis that focuses how the anaemia and signs and symptoms are affecting her ability to carry out the activities of living. The need statement identifies the activity of living that she cannot do (mobility – exhausted following activities and dizzy when standing from a sitting position) and confirms that there has been movement along the dependence–independence continuum (what she can and cannot do) caused by a physical influencing factor (the anaemia).

Sometimes, one or more of the 'problems' in the group can be included in the baseline and not the need statement. For example, we have not included 'breathless on exertion' and 'reduced sleep pattern and night sweats' in the need statement. This is because it would make the statement long and complex and Suzy didn't really see this as a main issue. These are, however, problems that have been identified from the assessing process and grouped together as a consequence of their being interrelated and interdependent, so we will need to include them in the baselines. This ensures that these problems will be reflected in the goal and intervention and therefore not forgotten. This is an example of how systematic diagnosis is a skill that takes knowledge and time to develop. A knowledgeable, experienced nurse would be able to make the decision that, in Suzy's case, being breathless on exertion and reduced sleep and night sweats will resolve once the anaemia has been dealt with.

The nursing diagnosis is confirmed by going back to the patient to clarify that the problems have been included in the need statement and that it represents their experience. When developing a nursing diagnosis (or any other argument), the final step is to check that the idea you produced during the synthesis stage is appropriate. In systematic nursing diagnosis, you need to share the diagnosis and need statements with the patient and engage in a conversation to ascertain whether the issues have been identified. Sometimes you will have to explain the thinking behind your decision to the patient and perhaps explain the nursing diagnosis that relates to potential problems or problems that they were not even aware of. You now have a firm basis on which to plan the goals and prescribe the care.

Systematic nursing diagnosis is a complex task that demands an ability to make use of thought processes at a high level. Trying to describe what you have to do in a step by step guide is not easy and on first reading you may feel really daunted and confused, but take heart, it will become easier. If I was to write down all the steps, movements and thoughts you have to engage in when you ride a bike it would be just as baffling, but getting on the bike and practising it makes it easier to understand. As you develop your skills and engage in critical thinking and analysis you will be able to apply these to your practice of care planning. In time you will find that being able to identify the problem and form a nursing diagnosis will become second nature, just like riding a bike.

Systematic nursing diagnosis using Orem's Model of Nursing

Orem is clear that nursing diagnosis is very different from medical diagnosis. For Orem, nursing diagnosis is the process that helps nurses to identify the patient's current therapeutic self-care deficits (problems) and whether there is the potential for future deficits. Orem cautioned the nurse to identify possible interaction between universal, developmental and health deviation self-care requisites (HDSCRs) at this stage. This interaction is illustrated in Practice example 8.1 in Chapter 8, where it was noted that there was considerable interaction between the USCR of sufficient intake of water and food, the developmental SCR of bereavement and the HDSCR of chest infection, as Albert was not eating a sufficient diet due to the death of his wife, making him more susceptible to infections.

At this stage the patient's needs or problems are identified from the assessment, along with the appropriate baselines. Remember that a baseline offers a description or measurement of where the patient is now in relation to the need. It provides information that will prove crucial in judging the patient's progress towards the identified goal during the ongoing and final evaluation stage.

Activity 9.3

Moire is a 47-year-old headmistress admitted to a secure mental health unit following serious concerns for her well-being being raised by her general practitioner. On admission to the unit, the assessment nurse produced the following needs statement:

Need statement: Bipolar disorder.

Consider the above need statement. Can you identify the limitations of this statement?

Have a look at Activity 9.3.

How did you get on with Activity 9.3? The main issue with the need statement is that it is a medical diagnosis: it is a health deviation self-care requisite that is the cause of a number of problems for Moire, and not a self-statement that has come from a nursing diagnosis. Nurses do not treat medical diagnoses but focus instead on the consequences that the medical diagnosis has on the lives of patients – in Moire's case, her inability to sleep, work or care for her personal hygiene as a result of having bipolar disorder. In addition, a need statement according to Orem, should wherever possible contain self-statements. These are statements using the patient's own words, usually (but not always) related to a USCR and conveying how self-caring the patient is. By using their own words, the patient will have ownership of the care process, making it more likely that they will understand, give their consent to and adhere to their plan of care.

In Activity 9.3, no baselines have been identified, making it more difficult to evaluate the care given in the ongoing and final evaluation stage of the ASPIRE process. As the statement in Activity 9.3 is simply a medical diagnosis, it is not specific to what the problem actually is and how it is affecting Moire's ability to be self-caring. It would therefore be difficult to prescribe nursing care to alleviate the problem and help Moire to return to being self-caring. Some important elements of nursing care may therefore be overlooked. Finally, the need statement does not state what the problem is due to, which means that the correct care to alleviate or solve the problem may not be selected. For example, difficulty in breathing can be due to asthma, chest infection, choking or a number of other causes, but the care to alleviate it will change depending upon its cause, it is therefore desirable to identify the cause of the problem in the need statement.

Moire's situation calls for more than one need statement to deal with her problems of living with bipolar disorder, an example of which could be: Moire says she cannot sleep properly, due to her bipolar disorder.

Baselines

+ Cannot fall to sleep, mind is racing, has not slept for 72 hours
+ Cannot concentrate on any tasks

Managing the other problems associated with the bipolar disorder will require additional need statements and baselines.

Identifying the relevant needs from the assessment is what systematic nursing diagnosis does. We have explored the difference between medical diagnosis and nursing diagnosis and how to write a need statement and baselines using the Activities of Living Model in the previous section. Now we will repeat this using Orem's Self-Care Model. To recap, when offering a medical diagnosis a doctor will often consider all the possible problems that arise from the signs and symptoms and offer a single diagnosis by reducing all the possibilities to the one thing that is causing the effect, usually a biological cause. Systematic nursing diagnosis is about establishing the problems that a patient has as a consequence of living with the signs and symptoms or the medical diagnosis.

This means that we have to start with the signs and symptoms or medical diagnosis and establish the nursing problems that originate from this label, this is a holistic approach. The list of signs and symptoms is usually long, because nursing care is about dealing with a patient's holistic needs. To add another level of complexity, you also need to recognise that many of these signs and symptoms will be interrelated and interdependent. Once again, the process of systematic nursing diagnosis that we are advocating allows you to make sense of these issues and ensure that you don't miss any key areas of need.

To help reinforce that process – and identify the links with Orem's model of self-care – let's work through the six stages of systematic nursing diagnosis, this time in relation to George Brown (our patient discussed in Appendix B).

First, a holistic and comprehensive assessment is conducted. You can see a full assessment in Appendix B. Next, analysis takes place and possible problems are identified. This is where we break down the assessment information into smaller parts and identify the key features. In practical terms, this means identifying and listing the actual and potential problems noted from the assessment. When using Orem's model, the problems are established by identifying a change in the patient's present routine when compared to their previous routines in relation to one or more of the universal self-care requisites; this change reflects the ability of the person to self-care, as a result of one or more causes.

Activity 9.4

Have a go at identifying all of George's problems from his assessment (Appendix B).

How did you get on with Activity 9.4? Your list of problems could look like this:

+ pain in ribs and lower back;
+ discomfort due to sore skin around anus;
+ skin around anus is red and dry;
+ frequency of bowel movements;
+ feels isolated and fed-up;
+ sleep disturbed;
+ not coping;
+ occasional urinary incontinence;
+ uncomfortable due to swollen testes and penis;
+ turning off hearing aid;
+ not socialising with family and friends;
+ weight loss;
+ reduced mobility;
+ potential problem of pressure sores developing;
+ potential breakdown of skin around genital area.

Once this list of problems have been identified, the third step of the systematic nursing diagnosis process requires you to establish how they relate to each other and how interdependent they are (see Table 9.2).

For example, George is at risk of developing pressure sores, but looking down the list using your skills of critical thinking allows you to see that the problems of weight loss, reduced mobility and occasional urinary incontinence are all related to the problem of developing a pressure sore. We should therefore group these interrelated problems together. George's problem of disturbed sleep is partly dependent on the pain in his ribs and lower back in the sense that if the pain is addressed, the sleep will improve – this is an example of problems that are interpendent. Equally turning off his hearing aid, does not feel like socialising and feeling fed-up and isolated need grouping together because they are interrelated (see Table 9.2). But if we prescribe interventions to help George with his pain and problems of incontinence, he will feel more able to socialise. His ability to socialise is dependent on the pain and incontinence and if these are dealt with George will feel more able to socialise.

Systematic Nursing Diagnosis is a skill that requires knowledge and experience to develop. A knowledgeable, experienced nurse would be able to make the decision as to which problems are interrelated and which ones are interdependent, so that the problems can be grouped together (see Table 9.2) .

Table 9.2 Systematic nursing diagnosis for George Brown

Self-care deficit

Pain in ribs and lower back	+ Pain in ribs and back + Sleep disturbed + Sleeps in a chair sometimes
Frequent loose stools	+ Frequent loose stools + States he is sore and uncomfortable + Area surrounding anus is red and dry + George is not coping with frequent bowel movements
Occasional problems 'holding his water'	+ Incontinent of urine 2–3 times a week + Has difficulty getting to the toilet at night + Passes urine 8–10 times a day
Uncomfortable due to swollen testes and penis	+ Pain in testes + Swollen testes and penis + Skin on scrotum pink, no breaks
Fed-up and isolated	+ Turns off hearing aid when family and friends visit + Does not feel like socialising + Feels isolated and fed-up
Risk of pressure sores	+ Has recently lost weight + Less mobile + Incontinent of urine + Skin around areas prone to pressure is free from redness and is intact

We're now in the position where we can move onto steps four and five of the process – using critical analysis to identify nursing diagnoses that reflect the consequences for George of living with his health issues and then synthesising that diagnosis into a set of clear, concise need statements and baselines. In George's case, we need to approach these steps with Orem's model in mind – in other words, we need to prioritise problems with George and use the key concepts of the model – self-care agency, Universal Self-Care Requisites (USCRs), Developmental Self-Care Requisites (DSCRs) and Health Deviation Self-Care Requisites (HDSCRs).

Consider the need statement from Appendix B: 'George states that he feels fed-up and isolated because of his recent illness, pain and incontinence.' This need statement reflects the nursing diagnosis for George or what it is like to live with the problems in the list. You will see that a self-statement has been used that conveys what the problem is for George in his own words, which directly relates to a USCR (balance between solitude and social activity). The need statement also includes some explanation of why George is feeling fed-up and isolated. The full extent of the problem can be judged by looking at George's previous social activity (documented in the assessment) with his baselines (where he is now). It can be deduced from the answers to the questions asked in the assessment that George's problems are likely to be caused by a change in behaviour and lack of motivation, arising from the medical diagnosis of cancer.

Sometimes, one or more of the problems that you identify can be included in the baseline and in a need statement. For example, we have not included 'turning off hearing aid when friends and family visit' in the need statement. This is because it would make the statement long and complex. It is, however, a problem that has been identified from the assessing process as being related to George's feelings of isolation, so we will need to include it in the baselines. This ensures that these problems will be reflected in the goal and intervention and therefore not forgotten.

The final stage of this process is where you share the diagnosis and need statements with the patient and ascertain whether the issues have been identified. Sometimes you will have to explain the thinking behind your decision to the patient. You now have a firm basis on which to plan the goals and prescribe the care.

Think about Activity 9.5.

Activity 9.5

Consider George Brown (Appendix B) and his lack of social interaction. Write a need statement that reflects the key concepts. Don't forget to include his baselines (a description of where the patient is now).

Compare your answer to the care plan in Appendix B, relating to need statement number 5.

Systematic nursing diagnosis using the Neuman Systems Model

As with all nursing models, Neuman's System Model (NSM) advocates using the assessment information to help you develop what is described as 'a clear, comprehensive statement of the client condition' (Neuman 2010b). To see how we can do this, let's have another look at Shoaib Hameed – our patient who has suffered a myocardial infarction.

You might remember that, by the end of the assessment, we had developed a summary of Shoaib's condition that was agreed between the patient and the nurse. If you need a reminder, the summary can be found in Appendix C.

Using the information from the assessment summary, we can set about developing some nursing diagnoses, need statements and baselines using the six-step approach that we've explored earlier. If you remember, we start with our comprehensive assessment, analyse the findings to list problems (those areas of concern to Shoaib and/or us), use critical thinking skills to identify which problems are interrelated and interdependent (and group them accordingly), develop a nursing diagnosis that reflects the impact of health problems on Shoaib, turn this into a series of need statements and baselines and then check with Shoaib that these reflect his concerns – easy!

You can see in Appendix C that we've listed a number of problems (Neuman prefers to use the term 'variance from wellness') that were identified in the assessment and then grouped those related and dependent issues together. One of these groupings is very clearly focused around anxiety, so one of our nursing diagnoses is going to be centred on Shoaib's feelings of anxiety.

However, anxiety is an extremely broad issue, so our nursing diagnosis and need statement also have to include some information about why he is anxious. Patients in hospital are anxious for all kinds of reasons: worries about their health, potential investigations or surgery, pain, concerns about their family, not liking the food – we could go on. You need to use what you know about the patient to rule out those things that are not contributing to the problem. For example, we know from our assessment that Shoaib is pain-free, and he has no major investigations pending. Our comprehensive assessment has given us lots of clues to what is causing his anxiety: using critical analysis skills can help us diagnose that he seems most concerned about the fact that he suffered a life-threatening event, that this may happen again, and that the heart attack will affect his future lifestyle.

That's a complex diagnosis, but we need to try and synthesise it into one clear need statement and associated baselines. These should sum up the problem and highlight the main factors. Try Activity 9.6.

Activity 9.6

Thinking about the problem discussed in the text related to Shoaib's anxiety, and try to write a one-sentence need statement that includes the reasons behind the problem. Also, provide some baselines related to this 'anxiety' need statement.

How did you get on with Activity 9.6? There are not really any right or wrong answers with this: as long as the need statement included the problem and the reasons behind it, then it will certainly serve the purpose. To save you a trip to Appendix C, here is the need statement that we came up with in relation to Shoaib: 'Shoaib is feeling extremely anxious because he is worried about his future health and lifestyle following his heart attack'. In terms of baselines, we've included some additional information in the form of:

+ On a scale of 0–10, Shoaib indicates that his 'worry' level is 8
+ Shoaib believes he will not be able to return to work, and will suffer financially as a result. He also believes that sexual relations with his wife may not be possible.

Of course, Shoaib has more problems than just his anxiety, so you need to complete Activity 9.7. Remember some of the tips that we've discussed earlier in the chapter. You can take all the issues that are of concern to you and Shoaib, and then organise them under 'umbrella' headings that will form your nursing diagnoses. You can then synthesise these into need statements and baselines that reflect Shoaib's thoughts, feelings and concerns. See how you get on.

Activity 9.7

Referring to Shoaib's assessment in Appendix C, systematically develop another three need statements and associated baselines. Once you have done this, have a look at the complete care plan to check your answers.

Once you have completed Activity 9.7, and had a look at the list of need statements and baselines that we came up with for Shoaib, we will be ready for the next stage of ASPIRE – planning care to deal with the problems.

Conclusion

This process of systematic nursing diagnosis is largely the same, regardless of which nursing model you use, but the need statements do look different. Using the Activities of Living Model will lead you to produce a list of actual and potential problems that include reference to the impact on activities of living and the influencing factors. Orem's Self-Care Model has a strong focus on 'self-statements', allowing the patient themselves to define the nursing diagnosis. The Neuman Systems Model helps you to identify 'variances from wellness' and use these in the nursing diagnosis. Whatever the process, the six-step process of systematic nursing diagnosis provides a springboard for the next stage, the planning of nursing care.

Chapter 10
Planning care

Why this chapter matters

Plans are crucial in all aspects of our lives. It may often happen subconsciously, and we certainly don't always write plans down, but we're often making plans in one form or another. One of the best places to watch people planning is during sporting events. Take football as an example: a team will go out and follow the plan that has been put together by the manager. This plan might be to play in a 4-4-2 or 4-5-1 formation; it might be to push forward or hold back; the players might have been told to tackle heavily or take it easy. During the match, each player will be formulating plans throughout the game. Some might be made in an instant – 'I'm going to pass the ball back to the goalkeeper' – while others might require a little more thought. Next time you watch a football match, just watch the player about to take a free kick from a dangerous position. Once they've done their in-depth assessment of how far away they are, where the wall is, where the wind is blowing from, they'll decide where and how they are going to take the kick. Without this plan, they'll never score: they'll just hit the ball vaguely towards the goal and hope for the best.

When you are caring for a patient, you don't want to be doing the nursing equivalent of kicking the ball in roughly the right direction and hoping it ends up in the net. You want to be sure that you, your colleagues and your patient can see how the care is going to be delivered. This chapter is one of the longest in the book, and that is because planning is arguably the most complicated stage of the problem-solving approach to care. This chapter will take you through the planning stage, step-by-step, from planning goals through to prescribing care in order to meet your goals.

By the end of this chapter you will be able to:

+ formulate goals that meet the PRODUCT criteria;
+ prescribe care in a clear, unambiguous way.

Planning using the Activities of Living Model

This stage involves the 'making of the care plan': the nurse identifies a goal and prescribes the care that will meet the identified needs. Remember, it is important to make the patient central to this process.

Setting goals

According to RLT the purpose of setting goals is to solve or alleviate problems and, where possible, avoid potential problems from becoming actual problems. As discussed, goals should offer a short, directive statement as to the outcome of the nursing care. If a base-line is where the patient is now in relation to the problem, then a goal represents where the patient should be as a result of the nursing care. RLT firmly believe that all goals should be realistic and achievable and must be set in partnership with the patient, and for reasons already discussed in Chapter 3, they prefer goals to be short term.

In Chapter 2 we mentioned that it may help you when you are writing a goal to consider the following:

+ Who is meant to achieve the goal?
+ What are they meant to achieve?
+ How are they meant to do it?
+ When are they to do it by?

We also introduced you to a set of criteria to compare your goals with. These PRODUCT criteria are summarised in Exhibit 10.1.

Patient-centred – is the goal tailored to the patient's needs?
Recordable – can you document the progress towards the goal?
Observable and measurable – can you evaluate the progress?
Directive – is it clear who, what, how and when?
Understandable and clear – is it written in a simple way?
Credible – can it be realistically achieved by the patient?
Time-related – when is the goal meant to be achieved?

Exhibit 10.1 The PRODUCT criteria for writing goals

The philosophy of RLT's Activity of Living Model suggests that goals should relate to how independent or dependent the patient is in relation to a specified activity of living (AL) and, as such, they should identify observable, measurable changes in the patient's ability to carry out that activity.

Sometimes, complementary goals may have to be set because goal setting for one AL may have consequences for planning in another. An example of a complementary goal for Suzy can be found in her care plan (see Appendix A). The need statement for problem 3 states that 'Suzy says she is not eating a well-balanced diet, due to lack of money and motivation, she has lost weight and is having problems opening her bowels.' One of the goals to address this problem is that 'Suzy will open her bowels once daily by 24.10.12', achieved by the interven-tion of Suzy taking an osmotic laxative as prescribed by her GP. However, in problem 5, Suzy states that she feels 'exhausted', has frequent headaches and feels dizzy when standing from a sitting position due to anaemia. The intervention identifies that her GP has prescribed an iron and vitamin supplement. This would probably cause a problem with the activity of elimi-nating, because **ferrous sulphate** can cause constipation. However, we don't have to include

Ferrous sulphate is a drug prescribed for the treatment of iron deficiency anaemia.

a goal or offer an intervention to address the problem, because we have included a relevant goal and intervention that will deal with the constipation in problem 3.

RLT describe how there is a need to consider the available resources before setting the goals because there may be a need for alternative strategies when resources are not available. It wouldn't be a good idea, for example, to set a goal that relied upon two nurses helping the patient when there is a staff shortage on the ward. Whilst this may sometimes present a dilemma for the nurse, it is important that informed choices are based on the available resources rather than the result of previous routines and rituals. To try to reinforce some of these points, let's have a look at an example of goal-setting in Activity 10.1.

Activity 10.1

Annie Laine is a 75-year-old woman who fell several weeks ago whilst going to the toilet during the night. She sustained a **laceration** to her left lower leg that she dressed herself with a bandage and a cream that she had in the cupboard. The laceration has now started to leak through the bandage; the fluid is dark green and smells offensive. The district nurse visits, assesses the wound and takes a **Doppler** reading. He offers a diagnosis of a **venous leg ulcer** and prescribes a suitable nursing intervention that includes a **four-layer bandage**.

The district nurse writes the following need statement and goal using the RLT Activities of Living Model:

Needs statement: Annie has a leg ulcer.
Goal: To promote healing.

Can you identify the strengths and limitations of this attempt?

The attempt at devising a goal in Activity 10.1 demonstrates the importance of conducting a comprehensive assessment, to identify the correct nursing diagnosis. The need statement offered by the district nurse is really a medical diagnosis. As previously discussed, this makes it more difficult to set a goal, because a medical diagnosis doesn't identify the

Laceration is a tear or jagged wound.

Doppler is a type of ultrasound test that enables practitioners to differentiate between venous and arterial leg ulcers.

Venous leg ulcer is a breakdown of skin in the leg, due to increased pressure in the veins of the lower leg.

Four-layer bandage is four separate bandages used as one dressing on the leg to provide compression that will enhance the healing of venous leg ulcers.

problems that arise as a consequence of living with the leg ulcer. It then becomes impossible to identify the correct goal if the problem isn't clear or related to the nursing diagnosis.

In order to reflect the philosophy of RLT, the need statement should have concentrated on identifying a clear, unambiguous description of Annie's nursing diagnosis. The goal would have been much easier to establish if the statement had outlined the activity of living that she cannot do because of the leg ulcer and included a baseline. For example, 'Annie has pain in the left lower leg due to a venous leg ulcer that is disrupting her sleep and ability to walk and stand.' This is once again an illustration of how the quality of each of the stages is related and dependent on the accuracy and clarity of the previous stage.

The goal in Activity 10.1 fails to offer a directive statement to describe the outcome of the nursing care. It is more of an aim or a declaration of where the nursing interventions should lead. This causes problems for the nurse trying to evaluate whether the patient has reached the goal; for example, if I asked you to go and evaluate the goal, how easy would it be? The chances are that you would find it very difficult to evaluate Annie's progress using the goal 'to promote healing'. This is because it doesn't offer clarification as to who is meant to achieve the goal, what they are meant to achieve, how they are meant to do it and when they are meant to do it by. It doesn't contain any of the elements of PRODUCT as discussed in Chapter 2 and summarised in Exhibit 10.1.

RLT suggest that goals should identify the measurable changes in Annie's independence level – in other words, what she can or cannot do in relation to the specified AL. An example of this would be 'Annie will sleep 5 hours in her own bed by 21.11.12.' This is why the elements contained in PRODUCT are so important, because using them will ensure that the goals are written to reflect identifiable, observable, measurable changes in the patient's ability to carry out that activity. The inclusion of a time element would ensure that the care is evaluated at the correct time interval. This is essential, as changes in the level of independence need to be recorded on a regular basis, because there is a chance that the intervention may be making the condition worse. Alternatively, if the treatment is healing the wound and making it easier for Annie to sleep, mobilise and care for herself, then positive feedback will encourage Annie to cooperate and continue with the plan of care.

The jargon used in the wording of the outcome ('to promote healing') would suggest that the district nurse failed to acknowledge that goals should be set in partnership with Annie. Once again, the likelihood of Annie feeling part of the care plan and contributing to the process is reduced if she cannot understand what she is 'meant to be doing or what she is meant to be achieving'. This raises legal, ethical and professional issues if a contractual agreement has not been made between the nurse and Annie as discussed in Chapter 1.

Now look at Activity 10.2.

Activity 10.2

Consider the scenario of Suzy Clarke in Appendix A. Can you identify a goal for Suzy and her problem of thrush using the philosophy of RLT? Remember to make use of the PRODUCT criteria.

Hopefully, your goal will meet all the PRODUCT criteria. Our suggestion for a goal would be: 'Suzy will be able to pass urine without pain by 20.10.12.' It is clear that this goal fulfils the criteria of PRODUCT in the sense that it is a **d**irective statement that is **p**atient-centred and tailored to Suzy's needs. This is because the goal was set in order to meet a problem that originated from a nursing diagnosis. Suzy says, 'I have pain when passing urine'; this is due to thrush. The outcome is **r**ecordable, **o**bservable and measurable, because the progress can be documented and evaluated in terms of whether she can pass the urine without pain, thus making use of quantitative and qualitative data obtained from Suzy. This makes the goal **u**nderstandable and clear to Suzy and other care providers, because it is evident what Suzy has to do to achieve the goal. It is also **c**redible because it is a realistic goal for Suzy to achieve within the time frame, if she takes the medication and follows the advice offered to her. Lastly, a **t**ime frame is offered to identify when the goal is meant to be achieved and to make sure that an evaluation of the progress is made. In conclusion, using the criteria of PRODUCT creates an outcome that can be evaluated in terms of Suzy's progress along the dependence–independence continuum, in relation to the activity of living – eliminating – with the provision for recheck and evaluation to take place and if needed the process of ASPIRE to begin again.

Prescribing the care

Once the goals have been identified and agreed between the nurse and patient, you will need to prescribe the nursing care based on research and evidence-based practice. The care is in the form of activities that the nurse, patient, family or other healthcare workers carry out to achieve the goals. Remember, the prescription offers a set of logically sequenced instructions that direct the actions of the patient and caregivers. The directions should direct the patient and carers as to who is to deliver the care, what they are meant to do, when they are meant to do it and where they are meant to do it (if needed). The nurse should also be able to offer an explanation as to why the care has been prescribed.

RLT believe that the aim of nursing care is to promote maximum independence. This could involve helping the patient to acquire, maintain or restore their independence in relation to their ability to carry out the AL. This may mean teaching someone to give themselves an injection of insulin following a diagnosis of diabetes (acquire), or making sure that a patient is able to carry out the activity of personal cleansing and dressing whilst they are in hospital (maintain) or helping someone to learn how to walk following a car accident (restore). Sometimes the aim of the nursing care will be to help the patient learn to cope with a permanent change in position on the dependence–independence continuum, meaning that they are now dependent on others to help them carry out the activity or to do it for them. Have a go at Activity 10.3.

Activity 10.3

Lily is five years old and has a temperature of 38.8 °C. Her face is hot to the touch but pale and she has a dry mouth and sore throat. She doesn't want to play with her toys because she has a headache and she is shivering; she is listless and tearful and says that all she wants to do is lie under her duvet on her bed because she is cold. The doctor has diagnosed an upper respiratory infection and has prescribed antibiotics, increased oral fluids and paracetamol. The nurse prescribes the nursing care using the RLT Activity of Living Model.

Interventions
1. Note and report any pyrexia to medical staff.
2. Give any prescribed medication for 48 hours and record effect.
3. Record temperature.
4. Use fan therapy and tepid sponging.

Can you identify the strengths and limitations of Lily's care plan?

How did you do with Activity 10.3? A limitation of the attempt is that it does not offer a logically sequenced set of instructions that can be carried out by the carers. It would have been better to start the prescription of care with the instruction 'Mum or nurse to take and record the temperature' and offer a clear direction as to when this needed to be done. This is because an understanding of the level of temperature is central in deciding whether to carry out the other interventions and therefore should be the start of the prescription.

The directions are not clear in terms of identifying who is to deliver the care, what they are meant to do, when they are meant to do it and where they are meant to do it. In addition, the nurse that prescribes the care is required to justify their choice of treatment by offering an explanation as to why the care is the best available option for that individual. Remember, the care that you prescribe is open to public, professional and legal scrutiny; this means that care should always be based on the best and most up-to-date evidence. The choice to use a fan and tepid sponging is not necessarily the best available care for a child with a fever and can actually disrupt the body's natural mechanisms for dealing with infection (El-Radhi, 2008).

The philosophy underpinning the Activities of Living Model suggests that the prescription of care should promote maximum independence, yet there is no mention of Lily or her mum in the directions. It is important that the care is organised around Lily's normal behaviours, because promoting independence is about building on existing routines. As RLT suggest, it is easier to modify existing behaviours than change or introduce new ones. Lily's mum knows Lily better than anyone and therefore it is mum that should be the one to carry out the care, in as normal a routine as possible.

RLT also propose that the care should involve seeking, preventing and comforting behaviours, performed by the patient and the nurse. In the prescription of care, there is no mention of making Lily comfortable, although there is an instruction to tepid sponge if appropriate. This is despite the fact there is no evidence that using tepid sponging or fan therapy is effective in reducing temperature. **Antipyretic** drugs such as Paracetamol are

An **antipyretic** is a substance that helps to reduce body temperature.

effective treatments on their own, with tepid sponging and fan therapy ineffective, unnecessary and often uncomfortable for the child (El-Radhi, 2008). The inclusion of mum and Lily in the prescription of care would without doubt promote behaviours that involve acquiring, maintaining and restoring independence in relation to the control of body temperature.

As nurses, RLT recommends that we assess the interventions/treatments prescribed or carried out by others so that the nursing care that arises from this input can be considered. The attempt identifies that the doctor has prescribed medication, but there is little direction offered to guide the carers. For example, the plan states that the prescribed medication should be given for 48 hours, but it does not clarify who should give the medication, when they should give it or when the 48 hours starts and finishes. Also, there are no instructions to deal with the potential problems arising from input of others, e.g. observing and monitoring vomiting, diarrhoea and rashes as a result of the undesirable side effects of the antibiotics.

Lastly, there are no instructions as to when the interventions should be evaluated. Although the goal may have offered a date for expected achievement, the carers need to know when they should evaluate the progress.

Have a go at Activity 10.4.

Activity 10.4

Consider the goals in the care plan for Suzy Clarke (Appendix A). Can you identify the goals that are aimed at Suzy acquiring, maintaining and restoring maximum independence?

How did you do with Activity 10.4? Your answers could have included:

+ acquiring independence – goals included in problems 2 and 3;
+ maintaining independence – goals included in problems 1, 2, 3, 4 and 5;
+ restoring independence – goals included in problems 2, 3, 4 and 5.

The explanations for these suggested answers are as follows. If we consider one of the goals from problem 2, 'Suzy will have arranged appointments with her academic supervisor, personal banker and student services by 20.10.12', it is clear that the focus is one of acquiring independence. The practice nurse is empowering Suzy, by helping her make an action plan to contact the people who will be able to help her with the problems. In problem 1, 'Suzy will be able to control her feelings of panic to an acceptable level of 2 by 31.10.12' is an example of a goal that maintains independence. Finally, in problem 2, the long-term goal 'Suzy will feel in control of the factors that are causing her to feel that she is "not coping" and "unsafe" by 19.12.12' offers an example of planning that focuses on restoring independence.

Planning using Orem's Model of Nursing

Orem did not use the term 'planning', but her stage of prescriptive operations equates to this stage. Orem identified this stage as specifying how nurses will meet the therapeutic self-care demands (alleviate or solve the problems) of the patient. It should be defined who is to meet the demand (the nurse, the patient or dependent care agent), whilst always pro-moting the development of self-care agency (encouraging the patient to be as self-caring or as independent as possible). Orem was clear that a holistic approach should be taken and that the total situation of the patient, the conditions and the circumstances of their life should be considered when planning care. This is in keeping with earlier discussions about how problems with one activity of living (when considering RLT) or USCR (when considering Orem) will often affect other activities or USCRs.

Planning involves the 'making of the care plan'; the nurse identifies a goal and prescribes the care that will meet the identified needs, taking care to keep the patient at the centre of the process. Orem emphasises that nurses are working closely with the patient and their families and the care that is planned should take into consideration what they are able and willing to do. The care prescribed at this stage is contractual in nature; that is, you must be able to carry out the care you have prescribed, with consideration of the available resources. There is no point in prescribing a nursing intervention if the patient is not willing to agree or if you do not have adequate resources to do it. This is especially relevant to pre-written core care plans or critical care pathways, because the care is standardised and the same for eve-ryone. This means that the care is not individualised and therefore instructions that are not relevant to specific individuals should be removed from the plan, with an explanation as to why this has been done.

Setting goals

The purpose of setting goals is to eradicate or reduce the self-care deficit and avoid poten-tial problems from becoming actual problems. Goals should offer a short directive statement as to the outcome of the nursing care; if a baseline is where the patient is now in relation to the problem, then a goal represents where the patient should be as a result of the nursing care. Patient-centred goals should be set using the criteria we have identified in PRODUCT (see Exhibit 10.1). Orem's goals of nursing relate to:

+ reducing the self-care demand to a level the patient is capable of meeting;
+ enabling the patient to increase their ability to meet the self-care demand;
+ enabling the patient's relatives/supporters to give dependent care when self-care is impossible;
+ continuing to promote development of self-care agency.

Remember, it may help you when you are writing a goal to consider the following:

+ Who is meant to achieve the goal?
+ What are they meant to achieve?
+ How are they meant to do it?
+ When are they to do it by?

It is suggested that goals should relate to how self-caring or not the patient is in relation to a specified USCR and, as such, they should identify observable, measurable changes in the patient's ability to carry out that activity. Unfortunately, these are times when problems cannot be solved and the goal becomes to alleviate the problem.

Now try Activity 10.5.

Activity 10.5

This is an example of a need statement and goal for a breathless patient, taken from a core care plan used in practice. Can you identify the strengths and limitations of this attempt?

Need statement: ... is short of breath and mildly **hypoxic**.
Goal; Will have a normal respiratory rate and normal gaseous exchange.

If you have looked through Chapter 9, you will have identified a number of problems with the need statement in Activity 10.5. The need statement isn't individualised, it is full of medical jargon that the patient would not recognise and it does not identify the problems that arise as a consequence of living with breathlessness – this makes it more difficult to set a goal. It then becomes impossible to identify the correct goal if the problem isn't clear or related to the nursing diagnosis. This is once again an illustration of how the quality of each of the stages is related and dependent on the accuracy and clarity of the previous stage.

What the need statement should do is identify the specific self-care deficit that exists for the patient. Orem's philosophy expects you to put the person at the centre of the care-planning process; one way of achieving this is by using the patient's own words wherever possible in the written care plan. So an appropriate need statement would be 'I just can't get my breath, I feel like I am going to die', due to an acute chest infection. The cause of the deficit is identified by the nursing staff in the second stage of obtaining the nursing history. This helps the nurse decide the prescription of care to meet the demand. In the example you will notice that there are no baselines added to the care plan; if we do not know where our starting point is, it will be more difficult to see if the patient is improving or deteriorating as a result of our care. The baselines that could have been added are:

+ the respiratory rate is 30 breaths per minute, shallow and irregular (depth and rhythm);
+ the amount of oxygen being delivered is 28 per cent, via a **Venturi mask;** oxygen saturation is 92 per cent;
+ the patient is sitting in bed and unable to walk about;
+ the patient's level of distress is 9 (measured on a scale of 1–10);
+ sputum is green and sticky, approximately 15 ml per hour;
+ sputum specimen positive to infective organism.

Hypoxic is having a low concentration of oxygen.

Venturi mask is a type of oxygen mask that provides a fixed rate of delivery.

163

Let's use PRODUCT to critique the goal in Activity 10.5. This is not **p**atient-centred, because the nurse has chosen to use medical jargon, rather than the patient's own language. The consequences of this would be that the patient may not feel ownership of the goal and there-fore would not necessarily know when they had achieved it. The jargon used in the wording of the outcome would suggest that the nurse failed to acknowledge that goals should be set in partnership with the patient. The likelihood of the patient feeling part of the care plan and contributing to the process is reduced if they cannot understand what they are meant to be doing or achieving. This raises legal, ethical and professional issues if a contractual agreement has not been made between the nurse and patient as discussed in Chapter 1, The patient should always be at the centre of the care-planning process and it should be done within a framework of informed consent.

The goal is not **r**ecordable, **o**bservable and measurable as it would be difficult to assess how you would know if they were nearly achieving 'a normal respiratory rate and normal gaseous exchange'. The word 'normal' is not a good word to use as a rule in goals, as what may appear to be normal for one patient or member of staff may be very different from another. That is why you should be identifying what is 'normal' for your patient in the assessment stage, to help you when you write goals that are achievable and realistic. It is not **d**irective because it is not written as an outcome in terms of reducing the demand or increasing the patient's capacity. What the patient is meant to achieve is not **u**nderstand-able and clear and when they are to achieve it is not specified; therefore, this goal is not **t**ime-related. The inclusion of a time element would ensure that the care is evaluated at the correct time interval. This is essential, as changes in the level of ability to be self-caring need to be recorded on a regular basis, because there is a chance that the intervention may be making the condition worse. Alternatively, if the treatment is making it easier for the patient to breathe and improving their oxygen levels, then positive feedback will encourage them to cooperate and continue with the plan of care.

An example of some goals that do conform to the PRODUCT criteria to address this self-care deficit would be as follows:

+ Albert (who) will take 20 breaths per minute (what), on 24 per cent oxygen via a Venturi mask (how), whilst sitting in bed (how), with an oxygen saturation of 95 per cent (what), by 14.00 hrs 24.11.12 (when).

+ Albert (who) will state that he feels less distressed and his score will be 4 or less (what) by 14.00 hrs, 24.11.12 (when).

+ Albert's (who) sputum will be clear of infection (what) by 29.11.12 (when).

These goals are **p**atient-centred, as they are tailored to the patient's needs and the patient would know when they had achieved their goal. This is because the goal was set in order to meet a problem that originated from a nursing diagnosis. They are **r**ecordable, **o**bserv-able and measurable, because the progress can be documented and evaluated. It would be easy to assess if the patient was moving towards the goal from the baseline (indicating that the patient is improving and moving back to self-care) or if the patient was moving away from the goal, indicating that the patient is deteriorating. This is because there are observ-able measurable things identified, for example the respiratory rate, the oxygen saturation and the distress score, thus making use of quantitative and qualitative data obtained from Albert. This makes the goals **u**nderstandable and clear to Albert and other care providers, because it is evident what Albert has to do to achieve the goals. Also it has been written in a simple way, with no jargon.

It is **d**irective: it identifies who, what, how (when applicable) and when they are meant to achieve the goal. It is realistic and achievable to **r**each this goal and a timescale for achievement it is specified, making it **c**redible. A **t**ime frame is offered to identify when the goal is meant to be achieved and to make sure that an evaluation of the progress is made. In conclusion, using the criteria of PRODUCT creates an outcome that can be evaluated in terms of Albert's progress in his ability to self-care in relation to the USCR – sufficient intake of air – with the provision for recheck and evaluation to take place and, if needed, the process of ASPIRE to begin again.

In terms of the goals of nursing care for Orem, the nurse would be increasing the patient's capacity to take in sufficient air, by giving oxygen and sitting the patient up. The therapeutic demand would be reduced by relieving the patient's distress, reducing his activity and giving antibiotics to reduce the bacterial infection.

Consider Activity 10.6.

Activity 10.6

Consider the scenario of George Brown (Appendix B). Can you identify a goal, or goals, using the philosophy of Orem, for the following need statement?

Need statement
George states that he has 'frequent loose stools' due to previous bowel surgery; he says 'I feel sore and uncomfortable.'

Baselines
+ Passes stools 6–8 times daily, watery, pale yellow, no pain or blood.
+ Area surrounding anus is red and dry, but skin unbroken.
+ Doesn't feel able to cope any more and states 'It is getting me down.'
+ Comfort scale 1–10: worst 9 best 6.

Remember to make use of PRODUCT when you write your goals.

How did you get on with writing some goals for Activity 10.6? We've taken our goals from Appendix B so that you can compare your answers.

+ George (patient-centred, identifies who) will state that his comfort score is 6 or less (observable, measurable changes in the ability to self-care, identifies what) by 23.11.12 (time-framed).

+ The area surrounding George's (who) anus will be free from redness and hydrated (observable changes, identifies what) by 23.11.12 (time-framed).

+ George (who) will state that he can cope (what) with the 'frequent bowel movements' (relates to a specific USCR) by 26.11.12 (time-framed).

These goals meet the criteria of PRODUCT and also link clearly with Orem's model. The goals are **p**atient-centred and have been set in partnership with George and Elsie. They are specific to George, and are about the individual. It is important that Elsie is included in this process as she will have responsibility for some of the care that will need to be undertaken to achieve the goal (the dependent-care agent). Elsie will also be supporting George with the nurse in achieving the goal. The goals are **r**ecordable, **o**bservable and measurable – for example, you can observe the state of George's skin and you can measure his comfort score. The goals also comply with Orem's model as they identify measurable changes in George's ability to self-care. They are **d**irective statements as to the outcome of nursing and dependent care and clearly identify who is to achieve the goals, what is meant to be achieved and by when. They are **u**nderstandable to George and Elsie as self-statements have been included and medical and nursing jargon has been avoided. This also means that George and Elsie will feel some ownership of the goals. They are **c**redible goals, and are realistic and achievable. For example, as it is unlikely that anything can be done to reduce the frequency of stools (it is due to having large amounts of bowel removed), the goal of the care in this case is to help George feel that he is able to cope again. Also the resources have been considered that will be needed to achieve the goals. They also relate to George regaining self-care in this USCR, consistent with Orem's philosophy.

Prescribing the care

Once the goals have been identified and agreed between the nurse and patient (and family, if appropriate), you will need to prescribe the nursing care based on research/evidence-based practice. The care is in the form of activities that the nurse, patient, family or other healthcare workers carry out to achieve the goals. Remember, the prescription offers a set of logically sequenced instructions that direct the actions of the patient and caregivers. The directions should direct the patient and carers as to who is to deliver the care, what they are meant to do, when they are meant to do it and where they are meant to do it (if needed). The nurse should also be able to offer an explanation as to why the care has been prescribed.

Orem wants patients to regain their ability to be self-caring and to overcome the therapeutic self-care demand or help them to positively adapt to it when it cannot be overcome. This will involve using one or more of the helping methods to assist the patient to regain self-care. The nurse needs to choose the most appropriate helping method. Examples of these could be feeding a patient via a nasogastric tube (acting for); helping a patient to take their medication (guiding and directing); helping a patient to use a Zimmer frame when walking (providing physical or psychological support); supporting a patient in making lifestyle changes, such as giving up smoking (providing and maintaining an environment that supports personal development); teaching a patient about their medication (teaching another). Sometimes the aim of the nursing care will be to help the patient learn to cope with a permanent change in their ability to self-care, which may mean that they will be dependent on others to help them or to do it for them.

Whichever helping method is used, the nurse will have to judge whether to use one or more of the three nursing systems: wholly compensatory, partly compensatory or supportive and/or educative. As Orem's goal is to promote self-care, the system with the least amount of input from others should be used. Care should be organised around the patient's normal behaviours and coping routines wherever possible. The prescription of other healthcare professionals will need to be considered, along with care that arises as a consequence of the treatments. Have a look at Practice example 10.1.

Practice example 10.1

Michaela, a nine-year-old girl with Down syndrome, needs supervising with her hygiene needs following an **appendicectomy**. A core care plan for hygiene needs is routinely used in the ward area, which identifies the self-care ability of the patient and the timing when carrying out hygiene needs. The core care plan has not been adapted for Michaela, despite quite detailed instructions about her hygiene needs being given during the nursing history. A nurse has been asked to encourage Michaela to clean her teeth, which according to the core care plan states that Michaela is self-caring. Whilst in the bathroom with the nurse, Michaela becomes extremely distressed, as the nurse has handed Michaela her toothbrush and asked her to clean her teeth.

Let's explore Practice example 10.1 in depth. The prescription of care should give sufficient detail about the patient's previous ability to self-care, information which is obtained during the assessment stage, so that the prescription of care results in as little disruption to their normal routine as possible. For people with learning disabilities it is essential for their well-being to adhere very closely to their usual routines. If this does not happen, they may become very distressed, because they cannot carry out their own care when they are used to doing so. Clearly a logically sequenced, detailed set of instructions was missing from the plan of care. Michaela has a very specific routine to follow when cleaning her teeth, which she does after eating her breakfast and lunch and at bedtime. The following is part of the prescription of care for Michaela:

+ Nurse to set timer (brought from home, kept in toilet bag) for two minutes, prior to cleaning teeth, following breakfast, lunch and at bedtime.
+ Nurse to help Michaela put 1 cm strawberry flavour toothpaste on to toothbrush, prior to cleaning teeth.
+ Nurse to place toothbrush in Michaela's left hand and stand on left-hand side, occasionally prompting her to continue brushing when cleaning her teeth.
+ Nurse to evaluate effectiveness of care using baselines and goals after each time teeth are cleaned.

Once all of these instructions are fulfilled (which describe as accurately as possible her usual routines for self-caring) Michaela can clean her own teeth, but without the nurse to provide psychological and physical support to Michaela her ability to be self-caring would be undermined. As the information was given to the nursing staff about these specific instructions during the nursing history for Michaela, they should have been added to the core care plan instructions. This example shows how information obtained during the nursing history is often required throughout the care-planning process and reinforces the need to carry out stage 1 of the nursing history for every USCR, even when a self-care deficit is not obvious.

Appendicectomy is surgical removal of the appendix.

Now try Activity 10.7.

Activity 10.7

Consider the goals and implementations in the care plan for George Brown (Appendix B). Can you identify one that is aimed at increasing capacity and one that reduces demand, and identify an example of where dependent care and nursing agency is used? You should also be able to clearly identify *who* is to do *what*, *when* they should be doing it and *where* (if appropriate).

Your answers to Activity 10.7 could have included:

+ increasing capacity − goals in problem 2, with George more able 'to cope';
+ reducing demands − goals in problem 6, with George's skin remaining intact;
+ dependent care agent − intervention 1(b): Elsie to apply Deep Heat;
+ nursing agency − intervention 3(d): nurse to supply urine bottles and continence pads.

An example to demonstrate that 'who, what, when and where (if appropriate)' would be intervention 1 (c): 'George (who) to assess his pain using the pain scale (what) in between the medication regime at 10.00 hrs, 16.00 hrs, 22.00 hrs (when) and record on the pain chart (what).'

By having clear instructions, everyone concerned with giving care knows what their responsibility is. Making George responsible for care that he can deliver helps him to maintain his ability to self-care, something that George identified as being important to him and something that is valued in Orem's Model of Nursing.

Planning using the Neuman Systems Model

The assessment of Shoaib that we did in Chapter 8, and the systematic nursing diagnosis process in Chapter 9, gave us a whole list of problems. We know, for example, that Shoaib has a rather unhealthy lifestyle that will increase his risk of having another myocardial infarction (MI). The problems and baselines that we identified in relation to this issue can be seen in Exhibit 10.2.

Problem

Without lifestyle modification, and an appropriate medication regime, Shoaib is at high risk of future cardiac events.

Baselines

(a) Shoaib smokes 30 cigarettes per day (recommendation is to give up entirely).

(b) Shoaib's BMI is 32 (recommended maximum is 25).

(c) Shoaib's total cholesterol is 6.4mmol (recommended is <4.0), LDL 4.3 mmol (recommended <2.0 mmol), HDL 1 mmol (recommended >1.15 mmol).

(d) Shoaib has been commenced on **aspirin**, **clopidogrel**, a **beta-blocker**, an **ACE inhibitor** and a **statin**.

Exhibit 10.2 Problems and baselines

For the bulk of this section, we'll focus on the problem in Exhibit 10.2, write some goals for our care and prescribe some nursing interventions that may help.

Setting goals

If you've read through the first two scenarios in this chapter, then you'll have recognised the importance of writing goals that are agreed by the patient and you, and that are clear and understandable. Just as a reminder, Exhibit 10.1 at the start of the chapter describes the PRODUCT criteria again.

With Shoaib's lifestyle, there are a lot of goals that could be written. You might need a goal related to smoking, one to cholesterol levels, one to stress and one to weight. Take a look at the examples that are provided in Activity 10.8 and have a think about how you would do them differently.

Activity 10.8

Read the examples below of goals that have been written for four elements of Shoaib's lifestyle. What is wrong with these goals and how would you write them differently? Use the PRODUCT criteria from Exhibit 10.1 to guide you.

1. Stop smoking.
2. Reduce cholesterol levels.
3. Be less stressed three months after discharge.
4. Lose three stone in weight within four weeks of discharge.

How did you get on with Activity 10.8? Each of the goals listed have some good things about them, but there are also a number of weaknesses. Goal number 1 certainly reflects something that Shoaib wants to do, so it is patient-centred. It also gives us some idea of what needs to be achieved – he has to give up smoking. However, goal number 1 doesn't give us any detail about *when* Shoaib should give up smoking – should he stop straight away, or gently work towards stopping some time in the next few years?

Aspirin and **Clopidogrel** are antiplatelet drugs used to reduce the tendency of the blood to clot.

A **beta-blocker** is a type of drug used to reduce the rate and strength of contraction of the heart.

ACE inhibitor is a type of drug often used to reduce blood pressure and ease the workload of the heart.

Statin is a type of drug used to lower cholesterol.

Goal number 2, to 'reduce cholesterol levels', also suffers from being too vague. What do we want to reduce cholesterol levels to? What is our timescale? Goal number 3 does provide us with a timescale for achievement, but is rather subjective and difficult to measure – how can we judge if Shoaib is 'less stressed'? This goal would be much better if it contained reference to an objective tool such as those discussed in Chapter 6.

Finally, there's goal number 4. Again, this does tick a number of the boxes – it is centred on Shoaib's needs, it is objective and measurable, and there is a timescale attached. The big problem here is one of realism: nobody is going to lose three stone in four weeks, so the goal is essentially unachievable. This is going to lead to Shoaib becoming disheartened about his prospects of losing weight, so he may disengage entirely from this aspect of his care plan.

We have set a number of goals related to Shoaib's lifestyle (see Exhibit 10.3). These goals may not be perfect – please feel free to critique them – but they hopefully deal with most of the issues addressed above and link clearly into the PRODUCT criteria.

1. Shoaib will give up smoking immediately.
2. Shoaib will plan to lose 12.7 kg (2 stone) in weight within 12 months (BMI to 28).
3. By six months post-discharge Shoaib's total cholesterol will decrease to 4.5mmol, and LDL cholesterol to 2.0mmol.
4. By 24.11.12, Shoaib will be able to explain the need for, and adhere to, his medication regime.

Exhibit 10.3 Goals

Most of the previous discussion hasn't really linked back to Neuman's model, and that's largely because Neuman doesn't talk very much about goal setting. Goals are mentioned in the description of how to implement the model, but no set criteria for how they should be written are included. One important thing to consider is that Neuman does suggest the importance of prioritising goals (as do Roper, Logan and Tierney – see earlier in the chapter). You might therefore argue that goals related to preventing and treating life-threatening complications are a much higher priority than dealing with Shoaib's anxiety. If this is the case, then the goals should be written in this order.

Prescribing care

Once goals have been written, the next step is to plan nursing interventions that will enable the patient to reach those goals. With Shoaib, we need to think about his clinical needs and the types of intervention that Neuman suggests nurses should provide.

Neuman talks in great depth about 'prevention-as-intervention', something that we touched upon in Chapter 5. She describes three types of prevention – primary, secondary and tertiary – that nurses can assist with. These may be terms that you have heard before, but be careful: Neuman's definition of some of these is rather different to how they are commonly used in British healthcare.

Primary prevention is the first type of prevention as intervention that nurses can deliver. It essentially involves any activity that prevents the patient becoming unwell in the first place, or (to use Neuman's own words) to 'protect the client system normal line of defence or usual wellness state by strengthening the flexible line of defence' (Neuman and Fawcett 2002, p. 25). You can do this in a whole host of ways, but the most obvious things related to primary prevention are interventions such as health promotion and patient education. For Shoaib, it's a bit too late for the primary prevention of myocardial infarction, because the problem has already occurred. However, we might be able to carry out primary prevention related to other aspects of his health. For example, providing education and support might prevent the onset of post-myocardial infarction depression.

STOP AND THINK

Think about a patient who you have looked after recently. What types of intervention have you planned and implemented that are designed to stop problems occurring in the first place? These are examples of what Neuman would call 'primary prevention as intervention'.

It will come as no surprise that, after primary prevention, Neuman describes secondary prevention as intervention. Things get a little bit complicated at this stage: many healthcare practitioners will define secondary prevention as the interventions that you carry out to stop a medical problem recurring. In Shoaib's case, this would comprise things like giving up smoking, eating a healthier diet and taking regular medication (Barrett 2006). Neuman, however, defines secondary prevention as the treatment of symptoms. If we are planning care for Shoaib using Neuman's model, we would therefore view secondary prevention as the acute management of his myocardial infarction, including pain relief and treatment with **percutaneous coronary intervention (PCI).**

Finally, Neuman explores tertiary prevention as intervention. This relates to returning a patient to 'wellness' following an illness. In Shoaib's case, this is therefore the health promotion, medical management and rehabilitation that he will need in the weeks and months following his myocardial infarction.

WHAT HAVE YOU LEARNT SO FAR?

Neuman describes prevention as intervention:

+ Primary prevention as intervention is designed to stop patients becoming unwell in the first place.
+ Secondary prevention as intervention is related to the treatment of symptoms.
+ Tertiary prevention as intervention is aimed at returning the patient to a state of wellness and preventing further illness.

Percutaneous coronary intervention is an invasive procedure used to increase blood flow through coronary arteries in patients with either acute or chronic coronary heart disease.

Neuman doesn't provide any fixed criteria for *how* to write down nursing interventions, so we can use the general principles outlined in Chapter 2 and earlier in this chapter. We need to ensure that any planned interventions clearly outline who is to carry out the care, what they have to do, when they have to do it, and maybe even why and where they need to do it. Only by including this amount of detail can a care plan become a useful tool.

In Chapter 2, we talked in depth about the need for clear instructions when prescribing care. This discussion highlighted how you need to be sure that other people can understand what you want them to do, and that you can account for any of the instructions that you write in a care plan. These issues can be considered by asking yourself two questions whenever you write a prescription for care:

+ If I was a bank/agency nurse, who had never worked here before and never met this patient, could I follow these instructions?

+ If I was asked to explain these instructions 12 months from now because of a complaint or inquest, could I do it?

Look at Activity 10.9.

Activity 10.9

Think about the 'lifestyle' goals related to Shoaib. Pick one of them – smoking, cholesterol, anxiety or weight – and write a nursing intervention or two to help meet the goal. Remember the need to include who, what, where, when and why, and to consider the two questions described above.

How did you do with Activity 10.9? We've included the lifestyle interventions from Shoaib's care plan in Exhibit 10.4 for you to check your answers against.

(a) Nursing team to refer Shoaib to community smoking cessation team on 23/11/12.
(b) Nursing team to refer Shoaib to a dietician for dietary advice on 23/11/12.
(c) Nursing team to discuss goals (a) to (c) with Shoaib and family prior to discharge to ensure ownership of targets.
(d) Nursing and medical team to discuss reasons for secondary prevention medication regime with Shoaib prior to discharge.
(e) Cardiac rehabilitation team to liaise with primary care practitioners prior to Shoaib's discharge to discuss targets.

Exhibit 10.4 Lifestyle intervention

When planning care using the NSM, the finished product will not vary that much from the plan you would develop with RLT or Orem's model. The goals should still be detailed, patient-focused and easy to evaluate. The nursing interventions should clearly specify who is going to carry out care, when it should be done, what should be done, why and where. There are some subtle differences: the focus with Neuman is much more on prevention as an intervention, with the idea of protecting patients against stressors providing an underlying principle.

Conclusion

The planning stage of ASPIRE gives you and your patient the opportunity to set out exactly where you want to get to and how to get there. Whether you are writing a care plan from scratch, or individualising a core care plan or care pathway, the production of goals and prescription of care is a fundamental nursing skill.

Whether you are using RLT, Orem or Neuman as a basis of your nursing care, the goals that you write should meet the PRODUCT criteria, and the care that you prescribe should be evidence-based and clearly documented. To go back to the football analogy at the start of this chapter, you want to make sure that your team has a clear vision of what you want them to achieve and how they can do it.

We've nearly reached the end of our journey through the ASPIRE approach to care. The next stage is the one that will probably take up most of your working day but only a small portion of this book – implementation.

Chapter 11
Implementation

Why this chapter matters

The previous chapters have addressed the ways in which you gather information from your patient, decide on what the problems might be, set goals and prescribe care. We can now move on to looking at the implementation or 'doing' part of the ASPIRE approach.

The actual implementation of care is obviously a crucial part of the process, and providing care will take up the majority of your working day. Ironically, however, it is the stage of ASPIRE that we take the least time to explore within the book. This is because the groundwork for implementation has been done in the assessment, systematic nursing diagnosis and planning stages. The implementation stage really involves following the instructions within the care plan to provide evidence-based care.

By the end of this chapter you will be able to:

+ describe how the implementation stage of ASPIRE relates to the Activities of Living, Self-Care and Neuman Systems models.

Implementation and the Activities of Living Model

RLT are a little vague about the principles that should guide the implementation or, in their words, nursing intervention. Their belief is that nurses are traditionally used to 'doing' and therefore leave it to you as the nurse to decide what is required in the intervention stage. However, they do argue that it is important that nurses' decision making is explicit and evidence-based and offer a range of actions that may be used to help the patient to meet the goals:

+ preventing behaviours – actions that reduce health risks and encourage health behaviours;
+ comforting behaviours – actions that make oneself or others feel better, including physical, psychological and social comfort;
+ seeking behaviours – activities that help gain knowledge or information that may benefit the patient's health status.

RLT also highlight how there is a need to provide treatments that have been prescribed by other members of the multidisciplinary team, such as doctors, physiotherapists, occupational therapists, counsellors etc. When any of these interventions affect the ability of the patient to carry out the AL, you will have to deliver care that helps them regain their independence. An example of this would be if a doctor sited an intravenous infusion. You would have to maintain the infusion but also deal with the nursing care that arose as a consequence of the patient not being able to carry out certain activities because of the presence of the infusion: maintaining a safe environment, eating and drinking, personal cleansing and dressing, mobilising and sleeping. In addition to this you would have to deal with any soreness or infection that arose as a consequence of the infusion.

During the implementation stage you are trying to help the patient to aquire, maintain or restore their maximum independence in carrying out the activity of living with your nursing interventions.

Have a go at Activity 11.1.

Activity 11.1

Sarah is a second-year student nurse on placement on a cardiology ward. She has been asked by the charge nurse to go and discharge a patient, Terry, who is due to go home having been diagnosed with heart failure. The plan of care states, amongst other things, that Terry must have his discharge medication given to him and the indications and side effects explained. Whilst Sarah is trying to do this, Terry asks whether any of his discharge medications will affect his sexual function. Sarah realises that she doesn't know the medication well enough to answer this question. She understands her role and responsibilities in relation to the administration of medicines (NMC, 2007) and the Standards of Conduct, Performance and Ethics (NMC, 2008), so hesitates as she is unsure what to do.

Think about the issues that were discussed in Chapter 2 and the philosophy of RLT. What actions should Sarah take?

Roper, Logan and Tierney (2000) propose that there is a need to provide treatments that have been prescribed by other members of the multidisciplinary team and this would include making sure that the patient receives his discharge drugs, understands how to take them and what the contraindications and possible side effects are. Consequently, Sarah, the nurse in Activity 11.1, was attempting to carry out care that should have been included in Terry's care plan. However, we offered a series of considerations that need to be thought about when carrying out the plan of care when we looked at the stages of ASPIRE in Chapter 2.

One of these considerations was the need to establish if the plan was clear and directive; another was to make sure that there are always adequate resources available to deliver the care. Much of the time in your working life you will need to follow instructions written by somebody else. It is important that you are clear on exactly what the healthcare practitioner who prescribed the care is asking you to do and that you can do it using the resources available to you.

In Activity 11.1, it was obvious that Sarah did not have the skills and knowledge to carry out the nursing interventions asked of her in the care plan and therefore should have refused to carry out the intervention. She was right not to try to answer Terry's question, because she did not know about the drugs and their possible side effects in relation to sexual function (NMC 2007). Remember, you are accountable for the care that you give, even if it was prescribed by someone else, and you should always be sure that the care is based on sound research or evidence (Buka 2008).

It was essential for Sarah to reassure Terry and explain to him that she would find out the answer to his question and get back to him as soon as she could. In this sense she would be engaging in comforting and seeking behaviours as suggested by RLT. It is at this point that Sarah should have acknowledged that the issue fell out of her scope of practice and was beyond her level of competence, referring Terry's question to her mentor, so that he could deal with it.

The mentor would then have to explain any possible side effects to Terry – including those related to sexual dysfunction – in a manner that acknowledged and maintained his privacy, dignity, cultural beliefs and individual differences. RLT would say that this is an example of the mentor engaging in comforting behaviours, by trying to reassure and support Terry with his concerns. Every effort should be made to offer Terry material or information to encourage him to engage in seeking behaviours to help him to understand his treatment and make an informed decision about his care. One final point to remember is that Sarah and her mentor would need to document the nursing intervention in the care plan in accordance with local policy and professional guidelines. This is something that was discussed in Chapter 1, and it is always worth remembering the basic rule of records and record keeping that 'if something wasn't written down, then it will be considered that it wasn't done' (NMC 2009a).

In conclusion, whatever model you use, it is crucial that your interventions are within your own capabilities, meet the individual needs of the patient, and are based upon the latest evidence. It is also vital that you assess the effects of your implementation and evaluate whether or not they were successful, seeking out support from others where necessary.

Now look at Activity 11.2.

Activity 11.2

Consider the care plan for Suzy Clarke in Appendix A. Can you identify the nursing needs that arise from the diagnosis of thrush and from the interventions prescribed by the doctor? List the activities of living that the diagnosis and treatment could have affected and identify the type of behaviour that you and Suzy need to engage in to deal with the problems.

How did you get on with Activity 11.2? Suzy's general practitioner diagnosed thrush as the underlying condition and prescribed medication to treat the infection. It is important to remember that each of the activities – preventing, seeking and comforting – is behaviour that both the nurse and the patient should engage in. Your answers could have included the following activities and behaviours:

+ Eating and drinking – the medication prescribed by the GP may make Suzy feel nauseous. Suzy could be encouraged to read the literature offered with the medication (seeking behaviours). You could advise Suzy of ways to deal with the feelings of nausea and reassure her that the signs and symptoms will pass (preventing and comforting behaviours).

+ Eliminating – Suzy has pain on passing urine. You could advise Suzy on how she can relieve the symptoms (preventing and comforting behaviours) and encourage her to try out the interventions that you are recommending, whilst offering her the evidence underpinning your suggestions (seeking, preventing and comforting behaviours).

+ Personal cleansing and dressing – you could advise Suzy about bathing, personal hygiene and trigger factors, to help prevent further attacks of thrush and help her deal with the discomfort (seeking, preventing and comforting behaviours). Suzy could put some of the interventions into action and read the literature that you offer her (comforting, seeking and preventing behaviours).

+ Controlling body temperature – there is a localised temperature increase due to the inflammation and infection. You could advise Suzy on how she can relieve the symptoms (preventing and comforting behaviours). Suzy could carry out the suggested interventions to try and alleviate the discomfort (comforting behaviours).

+ Expressing sexuality – you could advise Suzy that whilst she has signs and symptoms of thrush she should avoid sexual intercourse (preventing behaviours). Suzy may choose to follow this advice to avoid further damage and possible transmission of the infection. (Preventing and comforting behaviours.)

+ Maintaining a safe environment – Suzy could be encouraged to ask you questions and access literature and internet sources (preventing and seeking behaviours) in order to identify the possible factors that increase her risk of a future infections. You need to explain the medication, contraindications and side effects to Suzy (seeking). Suzy should be encouraged to ask questions if necessary and take the medication (seeking and comforting behaviours).

In all of these instances you and Suzy are trying to acquire, restore or maintain independence in carrying out the activities of living

Implementation and Orem's Model of Nursing

The implementation stage equates to what Orem called 'treatment operations'. Orem has identified that this involves using the knowledge and skills for practice and the five helping methods:

+ acting for or doing for another;
+ guiding and directing;
+ providing physical or psychological support;
+ providing and maintaining an environment that supports personal development;
+ teaching another;

and uses one of the three 'nursing systems':

+ wholly compensatory;
+ partly compensatory;
+ supportive-educative.

The care is complementary to that which the patient or dependent-care agent can achieve; the nurse acts in a variety of ways to make up for any deficits in capabilities.

Orem offers specific guidance as to what the nurses should be achieving with their care:

1. *Perform, regulate and assist with their performance the self-care tasks of patients.*

2. *Coordinate the performance of self-care tasks.*

3. *Help patients, their families and others establish an appropriate environment for daily living that supports the accomplishment of self-care, but also satisfies the patients' interest, talents and goals.*

4. *Guide, support or direct patients in their exercise, or withholding of their self-care agency.*

5. *Stimulate patients' interest in self-care by raising questions and promoting discussions of care problems and issues when conditions permit.*

6 *Support and guide patients in learning activities and provide cues for learning as well as instructional sessions.*

7. *Support and guide patients as they experience illness or disability and the effects of medical care measures. Continue this support as the patient experiences the need to engage in new activities of self-care, or needs to change their ways of meeting current self-care needs.*

(Orem 2001, pp.322–323)

In addition, there is a need to provide treatments that have been prescribed by others such as doctors, physiotherapists or occupational therapists. When these interventions affect the ability of the patient to be self-caring, you would have to deliver care that helped them regain their self-care ability. An example of this would be if a doctor prescribes bed rest for a patient. Their self-care ability in many of the USCRs will be altered and you would have to provide the nursing care that arises as a consequence of this: sufficient intake of water and food, satisfactory eliminative functions, activity balanced with rest and prevention of hazards. Think about Activity 11.3.

Activity 11.3

Consider the care plan for George Brown (Appendix B), focusing on problem number 5: 'George states that he feels 'fed-up and isolated' because of his recent illness, pain and incontinence'.

Can you identify the nursing systems that are used in the treatment operations? List the helping methods that are used to deal with the deficits.

How did you do with Activity 11.3? Your answers may have included the following:

5(a) By checking that George's hearing aid is switched on and by ensuring George is being supported to interact during conversations, Elsie and the nurse are trying to provide an environment that supports George's personal development. The nursing system used is partially compensatory.

(b) When the nurse offers reassurance, explanations and advice she is teaching and providing psychological support. The nursing system used is supportive-educative.

(c) By enabling George and Elsie to attend a luncheon club the nurse is providing an environment that supports personal development. The nursing system used is supportive-educative.

It can be seen that, although George is terminally ill, the care (treatment operations) that has been prescribed for George encourages self-care and dependent-care as much as possible. The supportive-educative nursing system is used the most. It is very important when implementing care that nurses do not take over for the patient and the family if they are capable of carrying out care for themselves, but they may need to be there to support and educate the patient and the family in order to make this happen. This is in line not only with the philosophy of Orem, but also with the NMC standards of conduct, performance and ethics (NMC 2008), namely that:

+ You must support people in caring for themselves to improve and maintain their health.
+ You must recognise and respect the contribution that people make to their own care and well-being.

Elsie expressed a strong need to look after George and had been doing so successfully. With the dependent-care agency provided by Elsie and his own self-care agency, George had been managing the therapeutic self-care demands placed upon him by his USCR and HDSCR up to that point; however, as further HDSCR, in the form of increased unresolved pain, which led to sleep deprivation added to the therapeutic self-care demand, nursing intervention became necessary.

In addition to specific things that need to be considered when using Orem's model, the basic principles that were identified in Chapter 2 when you are implementing care also need to be taken into account. They are as follows:

+ Is the care individualised and patient-centred?
+ Is the care, safe, legal and ethical?
+ Is the care based on evidence or research?
+ Are the resources available to deliver the care: knowledge, skills, staff and equipment?
+ Was dignity and respect for the patient maintained at all times?
+ Was consent obtained in order to carry out the plan of care?
+ Were the actions consistent with the prescribed care – in other words, did you follow the instructions accurately?
+ Did you communicate with the patient, their carers and your colleagues in an effective and considerate way about the care?
+ Were the actions documented in accordance with the relevant trust and professional guidelines and policies?

You will have noticed that a lot of these considerations relate to the prescription of care that you produced during the planning phase. This underlines the key message that this book is trying to deliver – a good care plan can help make your actual nursing care more effective.

Let's explore these basic principles in relationship to the implementation of care (treatment operations) for George in Appendix B.

The care was patient-centred, ensuring that George and Elsie were encouraged to be active in the care; for example, George assessed and recorded his pain. All of the care was written with George as the main focus. George's previous self-care routines were identified and incorporated into the plan.

George's care was delivered in a safe, legal and ethical manner, in that care was delivered by a first-level registered nurse with the appropriate skills and knowledge to carry out the care. Ethically, certain points in the care plan need to be highlighted. The long-term goal for the problem relating to pain was that 'George will state that he is pain-free at all times'. As George has a terminal illness where the pain levels may rise as the condition progresses, to expect a patient to be pain-free could be argued to be unrealistic. If this goal was not put in, then the psychological damage to the patient may actually increase the pain. Pain is not just a physical phenomenon; psychological and social influences will affect a patient's pain experience. Encouraging George to think that his pain will be totally relieved in the future may actually make this happen. If the goal was left out, then George might well become despondent, adding to the negative emotional effects of pain, which would ultimately increase the pain.

The care was based on evidence, a specific example being the application of Deep Heat™ by Elsie. Massaging the area around the pain with something that produces heat stimulates the A-beta nerve fibres overriding pain messages to the brain. Dignity and respect was maintained at all times; George was consulted in the care that was given and he maintained control of that care and the way in which it was administered. This was ensured by finding out George and Elsie's normal routines for carrying out self-care (when conducting a comprehensive and holistic assessment) and using this information to prescribe the treatment operations that matched his previous routines.

As the nurse wrote the plan of care with George and Elsie, they were both consulted at every stage and agreement was sought prior to each implementation. Consent and concordance to treatments and care will be more easily achieved if the care has been planned with the patient and dependent-care agent.

All the implementation was carried out according to the instructions. Had something needed to be omitted due to a change in circumstances for George, then in the ongoing evaluation a statement would have to be made detailing what had been omitted and why. It is as important to document what you have not done and why, as it is to record what you have done. It demonstrates a clear reason why something was not done, rather than it looking as though something had been missed or forgotten. This would be especially relevant if the care was audited or investigated at a later date for either professional or legal purposes.

Communication between the nurse, George and Elsie and the rest of the community team was good. George and Elsie understood the care being given and felt able to ask the nurse for help, advice and support. The written communication clearly demonstrates the care being given and its effectiveness. Finally, all actions were documented according to the NMC guidelines (NMC 2009a). Records were written at the time of care being given, accurate and comprehensive records were kept, the patient's views were included, and signatures and dates were entered.

STOP AND THINK

If you consider an episode of care that you have given, would you agree that you have abided by these basic principles of giving care? Where do you think that you could improve, or are you happy with every aspect of care that you have given?

Reflecting upon our past actions gives us a chance to identify what strengths and weaknesses we have. By doing this we can improve our future performance and become better and more effective nurses (Gimenez 2007; Schon 1987).

Have a look at Activity 11.4.

Activity 11.4

Esther, a 79-year-old woman with dementia, has returned to the ward following a small bowel resection. After about six hours she is conscious and is making a good recovery; her oxygen saturation is 92 per cent. One of the instructions in the care plan states that a post-operative wash should be given. The nurse goes to give her a wash and tries to change the theatre gown for Esther's own night wear. Esther is reluctant to do this and begins to become agitated and aggressive.

What do you think you would do if you were the nurse?

There are a number of different issues that you might have thought about in relation to the patient in Activity 11.4. Esther has dementia; it is very likely that her cognitive ability may be made worse by the low oxygen saturation, pain and possible disorientation due to the recent anaesthetic. As giving Esther a wash is not an essential but, rather, a desirable aspect of her care, it would probably be better to leave Esther (after checking and giving care appropriate to preventing pressure ulcers – essential care). If you force Esther to have care, then this is acting without consent. If you are going to omit care that has been prescribed in the planning phase, then it is essential to document why the care has not been given and any action taken as a result of this. It is also advisable and desirable to explain to any relatives why the care has not been given. It may be that you could enlist the help of the relatives to assist in giving care, if they are happy to do so, as Esther may be more used to them than the unfamiliar nurses. By the next morning Esther's oxygen levels will be increased, her pain will be controlled and the effects of the anaesthetic will be wearing off. It is quite possible that Esther will agree to having a wash now, having forgotten that she refused the night before. Also, due to the nature of dementia, patients are often better in the mornings before they become tired, making them more cooperative.

As you can see from the above example, although a clear prescription of the care needs to be given, nurses must have the skills and knowledge to adapt the care to changes in the situation and always act in the patient's best interests.

Implementation and the Neuman Systems Model

As with the RLT and Orem models of nursing, the Neuman Systems Model does not include much detail about exactly *how* nurses should implement their care. However, Neuman does discuss in some detail the concept of prevention as intervention. We touched on this in Chapter 5 and provided a bit more detail in Chapter 10, outlining how care can be broadly categorised into primary, secondary and tertiary prevention. To finish off this chapter, let's have a look at some of the practical steps that you can carry out when implementing prevention as intervention.

Primary prevention as intervention

If you remember from Chapter 10, primary prevention as intervention involves the nurse trying to prevent the patient from encountering a particular stressor. To do this, you usually need to know what the stressor is, so you can take steps to protect the patient from this. One simple example may be recognising that a patient is at risk of developing a pressure sore and providing them with a pressure-relieving mattress to reduce the risk of this happening. In the case of Shoaib Hameed, we are too late to apply primary prevention as intervention in relation to his myocardial infarction. However, have a go at Activity 11.5 to think about what steps could have been taken.

Activity 11.5

Think about the scenario for Shoaib Hameed. If Shoaib had attended a 'well-person' clinic three years before his myocardial infarction, what potential stressors might you have identified as a threat, and what primary prevention as intervention might you have implemented?

In Activity 11.5, the main physiological stressor that you would have identified in Shoaib would have been his risk of developing cardiovascular disease (CVD) – a term that incorporates coronary heart disease and stroke. You may have also identified possible potential psychosocial stressors, such as problems with his family relationships, but we'll leave them to one side for the time being.

In terms of the risk of CVD, there are a number of interventions that you might have suggested and that Neuman would advocate. Primary prevention as intervention usually has two purposes: to reduce the patient's chance of encountering the stressor (preventing CVD in Shoaib's case) or to strengthen their flexible line of defence to reduce the chance of a reaction (Neuman and Fawcett, 2010b). The latter of these is quite difficult to do in Shoaib's case: you can't easily reduce the reaction to CVD. However, you could have provided some education to Shoaib so that he recognised any symptoms early and sought help.

Most of the focus would be on trying to prevent Shoaib from developing CVD in the first place. This would require interventions based around health promotion and lifestyle modification – something very prominent in Neuman's model. In fact, you would implement the same types of lifestyle modification for Shoaib that are outlined in his care plan in Appendix C. The only real difference is timing and motivation. If you had seen Shoaib three years earlier, the interventions would have been an attempt to stop CVD developing, and the challenge would have been to convince him that he was at real risk. Three years on, lifestyle modification is too late to be viewed as primary prevention, but Shoaib will now be fully aware of the importance of making changes to his behaviour.

Secondary prevention as intervention

Chapter 10 highlights how the term 'secondary prevention' can be a little confusing: it can mean different things to different people. In the NSM, the goal of secondary prevention as intervention is the treatment of symptoms to protect the patient's basic structure. In essence, secondary prevention relates to the treatment of the underlying problem and support of the patient whilst they are unwell.

In Shoaib's case, much of the secondary prevention would have taken place in the acute stages of his myocardial infarction. Administration of oxygen, painkillers and percutaneous coronary intervention might here be viewed as secondary prevention interventions. At this later stage of his journey, there will still be some secondary prevention interventions to be carried out for Shoaib, such as the administration of laxatives for constipation or sleeping tablets for insomnia. However, at the point at which we first meet Shoaib, the focus of our care is moving towards tertiary prevention as intervention.

Tertiary prevention as intervention

The third of Neuman's intervention types – tertiary prevention – is focused on returning the patient to a state of wellness after treatment and trying to keep them that way. The easiest way to think of tertiary prevention in terms of the care you provide on a day-to-day basis is to link it to rehabilitation. In the case of Shoaib Hameed, the care plan in Appendix C demonstrates a whole host of tertiary prevention interventions. The medication that he has been prescribed is designed to stop another myocardial infarction; the referral to the cardiac rehabilitation nurse will facilitate an increase in his physical activity and a programme of education; the lifestyle changes that we are encouraging will reduce his risk of further problems.

It is important to remember that primary, secondary and tertiary prevention interventions can be carried out at the same time on the same patient. Have a go at the reflective exercise below to think about the different types of intervention that you provide. You'll probably realise that your approach to the patient was a combination of three types of intervention.

STOP AND THINK

Think about a patient you cared for at work recently. Reflect on the different nursing interventions that you carried out and identify whether they were primary, secondary or tertiary interventions.

Conclusion

None of the models covered in this book goes into any great depth on the type of inter-ventions to be carried out by nurses. RLT discuss the support of seeking, preventing and comforting behaviours. Orem provides the most discussion of implementation, describing the three systems (wholly compensatory, partly compensatory and educative-supportive) and a whole range of different helping methods. The Neuman Systems Model focuses on prevention as intervention, with primary, secondary and tertiary categories.

Whatever model you use, it is crucial that your interventions are within your own capabili-ties, meet the individual needs of the patient, and are based upon the latest evidence. It is also vital that you assess the effects of your implementation and evaluate whether or not they were successful. It is these processes of rechecking and evaluation that we move on to in the next, and final, chapter of the book.

Chapter 12
Rechecking and evaluation

Why this chapter matters

By this stage in the care-planning process, you have gone a long way to dealing with your patient's needs. You have carried out a comprehensive assessment, diagnosed the nursing needs, produced some goals using the PRODUCT criteria and planned and implemented your care. To complete the process of care planning and delivery, you have two more steps to complete – recheck and evaluation.

By the end of this chapter you will be able to:

+ identify the types of information that you may need in order to carry out the process of recheck;

+ carry out the stage of recheck using the scenarios in the chapter in relation to the Activities of Living, Self-Care and Neuman Systems models;

+ describe the differences between ongoing and final evaluation;

+ carry out ongoing and final evaluation using the scenarios in the chapter in relation to the Activities of Living, Self-Care and Neuman Systems models.

Recheck and evaluation using the Activities of Living Model

Recheck and evaluation

Before talking about RLT specifically, it's worth just recapping the general approach that you should take to evaluate your patients' progress. First, you need to gather data during the recheck stage. This allows you to describe and document a patient's progress to date in relation to specific elements of wellbeing. Secondly, you use this recheck data to support your ongoing evaluation of care. This ongoing evaluation involves comparing recheck data with baselines and goals to evaluate the patient's progress to date and the effectiveness of care (the process). Lastly – at a time specified in the prescription of care – you carry out a final evaluation (again using recheck data) of the outcome of care and the process followed.

According to RLT (2000), the patient's behaviours or ability to carry out the activities of living (ALs) should be the focus for the decisions made in these final stages. The baselines and goals established in the earlier stages of ASPIRE are used as criteria to assess whether there have been changes in the patient's dependence–independence level. Progress should be directly assessed by observation and measurement by you, but also by asking the patient for their account of their progress to date in the recheck stage. When there is a failure to move along the dependence–independence continuum in line with the goal, a joint reassessment should take place to allow redefinition of the problem and the setting of alternative goals. Remember that if the goals have been achieved within the time frame, there is still a need to establish whether the goals were too easy for the patient or whether they were relevant and did in fact meet the need. Look at Activity 12.1.

How did you get on with Activity 12.1? The account offered by the nurse didn't really evaluate Jon's progress in relation to him acquiring, maintaining and restoring his independence when eating his meals. The nurse should have carried out a final evaluation for all of the goals in turn. This involves considering the outcome in response to the prescribed care (process), at every meal time; this is in line with the timeframes identified in the goals. The recheck information – describing and documenting his progress to date – would involve the monitoring and recording of Jon's account of his experience and the carer's observations and monitoring of his ability to choose his meals, eating pattern and worry score. In relation to the Activities of Living Model, the final evaluation should have compared Jon's actual behaviours with the individual goals at each of the mealtimes, to establish whether there had been movement along the dependence–independence continuum in relation to the activity of eating and drinking.

However, the nurse cannot make an informed decision as to whether there has been movement towards or away from the goal without the use of baselines. Remember, a baseline is where Jon started at the time of the assessment and a goal is where Jon would like to be in relation to eating his meals after the prescribed intervention. Sometimes there is no difference between the baseline and the goal because it is a case of maintaining independence and this is the case with Jon, yet there was no mention of the baselines or degree of movement away or towards the goal in the nurse's evaluation. The nurse really needed to make a comment in relation to each of the goals, e.g. whether he managed to choose his meals, whether he was full at the end of his meal, and whether his worry score increased or decreased in this final evaluation.

It is obvious from the evaluation statement that Jon was not included in the recheck stage; Jon and his subjective appraisal should have been the focus for the decision making as to whether he had achieved the goals in the final evaluation. The evaluation should then have been documented, but again the nurse failed to write an account of Jon's personal experience of the mealtimes. There was no mention of what he ate, how he felt at the mealtimes, and whether it was a pleasant or traumatic experience; this makes the decision as to whether the goal had been met or not very difficult to make. The nurse's account does not identify Jon's perceptions of the influencing factors that moved him along the continuum towards dependence and prevented him from carrying out the activity of eating and drinking.

Activity 12.1

Jon is a 14-year-old boy who has cerebral palsy (athetoid), who is usually cared for at home by his mother. Jon's mother has had to go into hospital for a few days and this means that he has to go into respite care for a short time, as he cannot carry out all of the activities of living independently. One of the problems that the assessment highlighted is that Jon has difficulties feeding himself. He does get very anxious about this, which makes his lack of coordination worse. His mother is worried that he will refuse to eat his meals when he is staying at the unit because of the unfamiliar surroundings and differences in the care that he receives.

The nurse writes a need statement with baseline and sets goals that need to be evaluated on a daily basis. These are as follows.

Need statement
Jon says that he cannot manage to get his food on to the spoon to feed himself at mealtimes due to his cerebral palsy.

Baseline
+ Can choose own menu for each mealtime.
+ Can use right-handed spoon with built-up handle.
+ Cannot load the spoon with food but can use spoon to take the food from the plate to his mouth.
+ Worry score about feeding himself: 8 at worst and 2 at best on a scale of 1–10.

Goals
+ Jon will be able to choose a well-balanced meal of his choice at each mealtime.
+ Jon will be able to eat until he feels full after every meal.
+ Jon will state that his worry score is 2 or less at each meal time.

Evaluation
Jon slept well. He managed to dress and wash with assistance and then spent the day playing on his Xbox, interacting with the other residents and watching a DVD of his choice. Has not managed to eat very much today.

Consider the evaluation section of the care plan and identify the strengths and limitations of the approach.

A joint evaluation does not appear to have taken place, or if it has then the nurse has not documented the outcome in the care plan. There is a statement that suggests that the problem has got worse, an observation that is visible when the baseline is considered, but the nurse failed to provide an explanation as to why Jon is not eating as independently as he was on admission. Chapter 1 explores the legal, ethical and professional consequences of failure to document nursing actions or explanations as to why the care has not led to an improvement in the problem.

In conclusion, this narrow, brief report offered by the nurse didn't really offer a final evaluation of Jon's ability to carry out the activity of eating and drinking. What was recorded in the care plan was a very descriptive account of how Jon had spent his day, based on the nurse's perceptions, rather than an analysis of Jon's experience. With the use of the baselines, information gathered at the recheck stage and the goals, Jon and the nurse could have made a final evaluation as to whether he had maintained his independence in relation to eating and drinking. This final evaluation should have been a joint venture to allow the redefinition of the problem, the identification of the factors that have influenced the lack of progression towards the goal, and the setting of different goals if necessary.

Now try Activity 12.2.

Activity 12.2

Consider the care plan for Suzy Clarke in Appendix A. Can you complete the documentation for the consultations on 17.10.12 and 20.10.12 in relation to problems 1, 2 and 4? Your documentation should include recheck information, ongoing and final evaluations for the goals in relation to problems 1, 2 and 4.

How did you do? Your attempt should look something like this:

17.10.12 − 1(abcd); 2(a); 3(ac), 4(abcd). Can demonstrate breathing and relaxation techniques following teaching today.

20.10.12 − 1(abcd); 2(cd), 3(ade), 4(f), 5(abd)

+ *Suzy had a panic attack last night, panic rating 4, lasted 4 minutes, used breathing techniques which helped settle the panic and gave her 'some control' of the situation. Practised breathing techniques and discussed the process of classical conditioning during the visit*

+ *Suzy has made appointments as per plan; will attend first appointment on 22.10.12 with academic supervisor, 23.10.12 with student services has got plan of action ready to discuss with her. Suzy discussed rota and need to identify house rules with flatmates on 17.10.12, friends seem to accept need to change, have started task. Suzy's coping level is 6 today*

+ *Has completed 7 days of menu plans, meals reflect diet requirements. Bowels open today − still hard but no pain, mucus or blood. Had headache yesterday on waking pain score was 6, no pain today.*

+ *Has not yet completed budget plan, is waiting until she sees personal banker on 23.10.12.*

+ *No pain when passing urine since 19.10.12, comfort level now 1. Vagina still a little sore, but no discharge or odour*

The first thing to note about these attempts at recheck, ongoing and final evaluation is that the language is short and clipped. More like the style you would use to write a report than an academic assignment; this is not a problem because you need to communicate a lot of relevant information in the least amount of words.

The account on 20.10.12 involves critical thinking and analysis, rather than describing Suzy's situation. Whereas, in contrast, the account on the 17.10.12 is limited to recording the date, numbers and letters corresponding to the interventions in the care plan, and confirming that Suzy can carry out the breathing and relaxation techniques. The entry on 17.10.12 is an example of rechecking – measuring and documenting Suzy's current condition – and is all that is needed. However, you would also have to include a comment if care had not taken place or been refused or additional care that is not in the care plan had been given. The account on the 20.10.12 is much longer; this is because it offers both an ongoing and final evaluation of Suzy's progress in acquiring, maintaining and restoring independence in relation to the three problems.

Problem 1 required you to engage in an ongoing evaluation of Suzy's experience of living with her panic attacks, because the final evaluation dates were not until the 31.10.12 and 19.12.12. Ongoing evaluation involves making a decision about the patient's progress and the effectiveness of the prescription and implementation of care (process), by considering the baselines, goals and recheck information. The baseline is considered in relation to the information that has been gathered and documented in the recheck stage and then compared to the goal. A clinical decision is then made as to whether the prescribed care is to be continued or not. This may be because you can establish movement towards the goal, or alternatively there may be a change from the baseline that demonstrates deterioration, this would mean that the assessment process would be repeated, unless the change was anticipated and could be explained. Equally if there is a change from the baseline that demonstrates that the goal has been met before the stated time frame, the care could be discontinued, unless the change is only a temporary improvement and the treatment needs to be continued (see Chapter 3).

The statement in the entry for 20.10.12 highlights that Suzy was involved in the recheck and ongoing evaluation stage, because it was her subjective appraisals that became the focus for the decision making as to whether she had made progress towards the goals of dealing with her panic attacks. The information documented included a panic rating of 4. Although the accounts were brief, they did focus on evaluating Suzy's ability to carry out the activity of maintaining a safe environment, making a judgement as to whether she had acquired or restored independence in relation to this activity that she was struggling to carry out. A clinical decision was made to continue with the prescribed care because movement towards the goal could be established as the baseline panic rating was 9 at worst and 5 at best. There was no unnecessary description of what care had been carried out, because this can complicate the read, making it difficult for anyone wanting to read the care plan to gain an understanding of the progress to date or whether Suzy had reached her goal. It is enough to write the problem number and letter that corresponds to the specific intervention, e.g. '1acdef'.

Your attempt at the task should have involved you carrying out a final evaluation in relation to problems 2 and 4, as instructed in the care plan (see goal dates for problem 2 and 4 and intervention 2d and 4f). In order to carry out a final evaluation, a registered nurse needs to consider the baseline, goal and recheck information on the date set during the planning stage and evaluate whether the goal has been achieved by the patient. In doing this they are evaluating both the process of care and the outcome. In other words, the question being answered is 'Has the care been effective in allowing the patient to achieve their goal?' Suzy's actual behaviours are compared to the individual goals, in order to establish whether there has been movement along the dependence–independence continuum. Reference to the baselines allows a decision to be made as to whether there has been movement towards or away from the goal. The goals for making the appointments with the academic supervisor, personal banker and student support and passing urine without pain were achieved and a discontinued date would be added to the margin of the care plan to indicate this. A statement as to why Suzy has not started the budget plan and what she intended to do to make sure the goal was still achievable was recorded in the care plan and the goal date for this particular problem was extended by one week.

When all of the goals have been met or when completing the discharge plan, it is time to establish whether the set goals were realistic and relevant and whether the prescribed care was appropriate in terms of meeting the goals. Issues of documentation and record keeping in relation to the patient's progress are considered, as well as consideration of the effectiveness of the Activities of Living Model in meeting the individualised needs of the patient and restoring their independence. This means that the episode of care has been evaluated in terms of outcome and in relation to the patient experience. Considering the ongoing and final evaluations for a variety of patients will allow you to see if the framework did in fact 'tackle the job'; that is, whether the problems were identified and dealt with effectively in a way that was clear and understood by the patient and whether the patient experience was satisfactory. Now have a go at Activity 12.3.

Activity 12.3

Have one last look at the scenario and care plan for Suzy Clarke in Appendix A. Consider the philosophy put forward by RLT. Do you think that the choice to use the Activities of Living Model helped the practice nurse plan the best available care for her and would you use this model for Suzy? If not, why not? List the strengths and limitations of using RLTs' Activities of Living Model for a patient such as Suzy.

Once you've had a think about the strengths and limitations of the RLT model, go back to the end of Chapter 3 to remind yourself of some of the published thoughts on the model.

Evaluation using Orem's Model of Nursing

Orem does not use the term 'evaluation', but the last stage of Orem's treatment operations, and something she calls control operations, equates to what we call ongoing evaluation.

At this stage Orem wants nurses to find out if the self-care deficits have been addressed. This would involve considering whether a balance between self-care ability and self-care demand has been achieved in a way that is acceptable to the patient. Once the relevant information has been gathered through the recheck stage, evaluation of a patient's progress can be made with reference to the patient's ability to carry out self-care. The baselines and goals that have been identified in the earlier stages of ASPIRE are used as criteria to assess whether there have been changes in the patient's self-care abilities. Progress should be directly assessed by observation and measurement by you, but also by asking the patient for their account of their current condition in the recheck stage. Remember that if the goals have been achieved within the time frame, there is still a need to establish whether the goals were too easy for the patient or whether they were relevant and did in fact meet the need. When there is a failure to restore the patient's self-care ability in line with the goal, a joint reassessment should take place to allow redefinition of the problem and the setting of alternative goals. It is also important to remember, as discussed in Chapter 2, that if the goals have been achieved within the designated time frame, there is still a need to establish whether the goals were too easy for the patient, or whether they were relevant to the patient's needs.

Evaluation involves making nursing judgements about the patient's progress in addressing the self-care demand. The patient's account of their experiences should be included wherever possible to keep the patient at the centre of the process. A return to self-caring should be seen as a sign of success – termed as recovery. As in the implementation stage, Orem is quite prescriptive about the behaviours nurses should engage in, to recheck and evaluate the care that has been given.

1. Monitor patients and assist patients to monitor themselves to determine if self-care measures were effectively performed and to determine the effects of self-care and the efficiency of nursing actions directed to these ends.

2. Make judgements about the sufficiency and efficiency of self-care, the patient's ability to regulate and develop self-care agency, and nursing assistance.

3. Make judgements about the meaning of the results of the above and make adjustments in the nursing care system through changes in nurse and patient roles.

(Adapted from Orem 2001, p.323)

In other words, how effective have the patient (using self-care agency), the family (using dependent-care agency) and the nurse (using nursing agency) been in achieving the goals set out in the planning stage? The purpose of ongoing and final evaluation is to see whether the patient has progressed towards, moved away from, or achieved, the set goal. This highlights the importance of identifying baselines and writing clear goals that you can use to evaluate the patient's progress. You cannot make an informed decision as to whether the patient has moved towards or away from their goal unless you have a clear starting point. Without a baseline, the best you can do is comment when the patient has actually achieved the goal. With the help of baselines, you can make a judgement as to the progress that the patient has made. The use of self-statements in the evaluation is useful to ensure that you get the patient's perspective of their evaluation of the care. Once these judgements have been made, the nursing systems can be adjusted. For example, a patient may have originally required partially compensatory care to help them overcome a self-care deficit; as the balance is restored by either reducing the self-care demand or increasing their capacity, the patient may only require support or education in the next phase of their care.

To help you to evaluate using Orem's model, certain criteria need to be considered. There should be clear evidence to demonstrate movement towards or away from the goal, with much of this information collected during the recheck phase. Behaviours or activities and the patient's personal accounts of their experiences should be the focus for the decision making in ongoing and final evaluation. Baselines and goals are used to establish the move towards restoring self-care, exploring whether the capacity of the patient has been increased (or the demand has been reduced) in order for the patient to cope with the deficit. If the goals have been achieved, it's important to ensure that they were not too easy and that meeting them is dealing with the identified deficit. If the goals have not been achieved in the desired time, then there may be a need to start the ASPIRE process again.

Let's consider need statement number 5 from George's care plan (Appendix B) to explore whether these factors have been considered when evaluating George's care. To do this we need to look at the evaluations and compare them with the need statement, baselines, goals and interventions (Exhibit 12.1).

Need statement 5
George states that he feels 'fed-up and isolated' because of his recent illness, pain and incontinence.

Baselines
Turning hearing aid off when friends and family visit.
'I don't feel like mixing with anyone right now.'
Fed-up scale 0–10, 9 at worst 2 at best

Goals (prescriptive operations)
Short term:
+ George will state that his feelings of being 'isolated and fed-up' will be 2 or less by 26.11.12
+ George will meet with his friends and family with his hearing aid switched on by 26.11.12
Long term:
+ George will be free from the factors that make him feel isolated and rejoin the social activities of his choosing by 19.12.12

Interventions (treatment operations)
5(a) Nurse/Elsie to check hearing aid is switched on, speak slowly and clearly facing George during all communications/interactions.
 (b) Nurse to offer reassurance, explanations and advice to Elsie and George, where appropriate, to alleviate anxious feelings or worries.
 (c) George/Elsie to attend Age Concern luncheon club on Wednesdays and Fridays – nurse to arrange sitter when George cannot attend.
 (d) Nurse to discuss the effectiveness of 5(a,b,c) at each visit using baselines and record (Recheck)
 (e) Nurse to evaluate using goals and baseline on 26.11.12 and 19.12.12 and record (Final Evaluation)

Ongoing and final evaluation (treatment and control operations)
20.11.12
Problem 5
(a, b, d)   Elsie states 'George is still not switching on his hearing aid, we don't seem to have moved forward very much.' Fed-up score unchanged from baseline, 9. Reassured that the new care measures will take 24–48 hours to start taking effect.

21.11.12
(a, b, c, d)   Elsie has enjoyed luncheon club today: 'I felt as though I could relax for the first time for weeks, knowing that someone was looking after George for me.' George slept whilst the sitter was there. He has not communicated with his friends or family today. Fed-up score 8.

22.11.12
(a, b, d)   George switched on his hearing aid during a visit from his son.
23.11.12
(a, b, c, d)   Elsie enjoyed luncheon club. George had a chat with the sitter with his hearing aid switched on, he said it was good to talk to someone distanced from his situation. Fed-up score 5.

▶

24.11.12	
(a, b, d)	George had his hearing aid switched on during a visit from a friend.
25.11.12	
(a, b, d)	George had his hearing aid switched on during visits from his son and grand-children. He played cards with his grandchildren for 30 minutes, which Elsie was very pleased about.
26.11.12	
(a, b, d, e)	George has his hearing aid switched on for most of the day and is meeting with and talking to his friends and family. He states 'I am less fed-up with myself, about a 3, I feel more sociable now that I feel more comfortable and less tired.'

Exhibit 12.1 Need statement, goals, prescribed care and evaluation for George Brown

The evaluation in Exhibit 12.1 shows how we can establish movement towards or away from the goal, using the process of ongoing evaluation. We can see that on 20.11.12 the care interventions that took place were recorded by using the appropriate numbers and letters corresponding to those identified on the care plan. Also on 20.11.12, Elsie identified that there did not seem to be much progress being made and this was of concern to her. To reassure Elsie and George, explanations were given to try to alleviate their concerns and worries, as suggested in intervention 5 (b). At this stage a recheck on George's 'fed-up' scale was done and no difference was identified from the baselines. This established that the self-care deficit (problem) was not getting worse and, as expected at this time, was not getting better either. In George's case, it was anticipated that the care measures that were put in place to alleviate George's problems and return him to being self-caring would take a few days to start taking effect and this was explained to George and Elsie in an attempt to reassure them. Consequently, even though the ongoing evaluation initially demonstrated no improvement, no changes to the plan of care (process) were made.

On subsequent days 21.11.12–25.11.12, all of the care given was recorded using the numbers and letters corresponding to those identified on the care plan, and ongoing evaluation was done which included the recheck information relating to George's score on the 'fed-up' scale. As there was clear evidence that the care measures were working, in that there was movement towards the goals, for example the 'fed-up' score was improving and Elsie and George's behaviours indicated positive progress, no changes to the care plan were needed.

On 26.11.12 a final evaluation is made in line with instruction 5 (e). The purpose of final evaluation is to see whether the patient has achieved the goal on the date identified in the planning stage and whether the experience was right for them as an individual. This requires the registered nurse to consider the information that they have available to them from the recheck stage and make a judgement as to whether the patient has met the prescribed goal(s). On 26.11.12 when the final evaluation was carried out with George, there was a clear movement towards the goals from the baselines as can be seen from the objective information – the fed-up scale score – and subjective information – George and Elsie's own words and views which helped the evaluation. The behaviour of George and his personal accounts – 'I am less fed-up with myself, about a 3, I feel more sociable now that I feel more comfortable and less tired' – are the focus of the decision making. Actual behaviours are compared with the goals to establish a return to self-care; for example, George is turning his hearing aid on and talking to friends and family. Baselines and goals have been used to establish that George is moving towards self-care in this universal self-care requisite of balance between solitude and social interaction. The patient's views and opinions have been included in the evaluation and this is important in view of the findings of the Ombudsman, which often suggests that patient's subjective views are not included in evaluations (see Chapter 1). Despite this progress, the final evaluation shows us that George has not quite met the short-term goal of a 'fed-up' score of 2 by the 26.11.12. However, George has made such good progress that no alterations to the care plan need to be made at this stage, except to extend the goal date. George's self-statement also demonstrates how interrelated and interdependent the whole process is. He states that he is feeling more sociable due to feeling more comfortable and less tired, aspects of care that are being dealt with under other need statements. By increasing George's capacity to cope with the self-care deficit, it is actually promoting self-care.

Remember that final evaluation is not just about ascertaining whether or not the goals have been reached. We also need to look at the overall patient (and carer) experience, whether the goals were appropriate in the first place, and whether our general approach to care was appropriate. Issues of documentation and record keeping in relation to the patient's progress are considered, as well as consideration of the effectiveness of Orem's model in meeting the individualised needs of the patient and restoring them to self-care. Considering the ongoing and final evaluations for a variety of patients will allow you to see if the framework did work; that is, whether the problems were identified and dealt with effectively in a way that was clear and understood by the patient and whether the patient experience was satisfactory. You should also be able to analyse how effective the framework has been in organising the delivery of nursing; utilising resources; restoring patients to self-care; or addressing their self-care deficits when self-care is not possible. Orem saw the role of the nurse as complementary to that of the patient and other healthcare workers and suggested that this should also be evaluated. During evaluation Orem was interested in identifying the nursing systems that have been used, with the emphasis on ensuring that the least intrusive system has been utilised at all times. This type of evaluation usually takes place after a model has been used over a period of time, with several patients. Areas that need to be explored include whether the model provided a framework by which effective care can be planned and delivered. This could include considering whether the model directed the care-planning process by being easy to use by the healthcare team. However, it is important to remember that the patient should be central to the process and therefore the quality of their experience is as important as achieving the outcomes, when conducting an evaluation. For example, a patient may have had a hip replacement carried out with a successful outcome, but the experience of the stay in hospital may have been so poor that the patient is fearful of future admissions. This means that evaluation is about establishing whether the correct model was selected for the clinical area, one that offers the nursing specialty the right guidance but also suits the needs of the patient.

Have a look at Activity 12.4.

Activity 12.4

Consider the scenario and care plan for George in Appendix B. Do you think that the choice to use Orem's model helped the nurse plan the best available care for George and would you use this model? List the reasons why you would use the model (the strengths) and list the reasons why you would not use the model (the limitations).

Once you've done this, refer to the discussion of strengths and limitations of Orem's model at the end of Chapter 4. You may also have found some more of your own.

Evaluation using the Neuman Systems Model

Of the three nursing models that we have looked at within this book, Neuman's model gives the least time to discussing the need to recheck the patient's progress and evaluate whether interventions were successful. Because of this, rechecking and evaluation using Neuman's model is largely driven by the general rules discussed in Chapter 2.

In other words, we need to look back at the baselines that we have recorded for our patients, look at the goals that were set, and decide whether or not the patient has progressed towards meeting the goals. This decision will be made by gathering appropriate data through rechecking the patient's condition, and comparing this data with the baselines and desired goals. Remember that, with Neuman's model, the goals of interventions are generally categorised as either to prevent the patient being exposed to a problem or to reduce the reaction to it (primary prevention), supporting the patient and treating symptoms whilst they are unwell (secondary prevention) and returning the patient to their usual state of well-being (tertiary prevention). These are the types of results you would therefore be looking for when evaluating a patient's care using Neuman's model.

Let's have one last visit to the care of Shoaib Hameed, our patient who has suffered a myocardial infarction. Have a go at Activity 12.5 to see if you can identify how you would recheck and evaluate his progress.

Activity 12.5

Because Shoaib has suffered a myocardial infarction, he is at risk of a range of side effects. In his full care plan (Appendix C), we've highlighted this as a problem, and written a goal in relation to it:

Shoaib will remain free of the following throughout his hospital stay:

+ chest pain or discomfort;
+ cardiac arrhythmias;
+ signs and symptoms of heart failure;
+ bleeding.

How would you recheck and evaluate Shoaib's progress in relation to this goal?

How did you get on with Activity 12.5? In terms of activities to recheck Shoaib's progress, there will be a variety of things you can do, including recording his vital signs at designated times, checking his stools for any blood and asking him how he feels – the whole list of suggestions for monitoring progress towards the goals can be found in Appendix C. By rechecking Shoaib using these techniques, you can produce a clear, focused report on his progress in relation to each goal. In our care plan, in relation to the risk of complications, the report for one day reads as follows:

+ Shoaib has not reported breathlessness, dizziness, or pain of any sort (0 on visual analogue scale).

+ Vital signs have remained within normal parameters throughout the day – values at 14.00 were blood pressure 120/70mmHg, pulse 70 bpm, respiratory rate 12 breaths per minute.

+ Bowels opened – no faecal occult blood detected. Nil abnormal detected in dipstick of urine.

Remember that there are two components to evaluation. First, we use information from the recheck phase to allow ongoing evaluation of the progress to date and of the effectiveness of prescribed care. By looking at Shoaib's current condition and comparing this to baselines and goals, we will have an ongoing picture of whether he is making progress. The ongoing nature of this evaluation allows us to identify a lack of progress or deterioration and intervene quickly. Then – at dates set out in our goals – we carry out a final evaluation to see if goals have been achieved, to judge whether the goals were appropriate, and to explore whether the process of care was effective.

One crucial thing to remember is that the methods and times of rechecking and evaluation are documented clearly in the care plan. For example, if you are prescribing nursing care to help with healing a wound, then part of your prescription of care must contain instructions on how often to measure the size of the wound to evaluate progress. This clear communication is particularly important for a patient like Shoaib, for whom much of the rechecking and evaluation will take place *after* he has been discharged. It will be his cardiologist, general practitioner and practice nurse who will be evaluating much of his progress in the weeks and months to come, so they need to know exactly what to be looking out for. Now try Activity 12.6.

Activity 12.6

As part of Shoaib's final evaluation, consider the framework of care used. What aspects of Neuman's model do you think worked well, and what were the weaknesses of the approach?

Once you've had a think about the strengths and limitations of the model, have a look at the end of Chapter 5 to remind yourself of our views on Neuman's approach.

Conclusion

This chapter has discussed the final two stages of the ASPIRE approach to care – rechecking and evaluation. Although they have been discussed within one chapter because of their close affiliation, it's important to remember that they are very different processes:

+ Rechecking is the targeted gathering of information and the describing and documenting of progress to date.

+ Evaluation is the analytical process (based upon the information gathered during rechecking) that you carry out to decide whether the patient is making progress (ongoing evaluation) and whether goals have been achieved or not (final evaluation).

Although the three nursing models used in this book don't talk a great deal about evaluation, it is a vital part of any care-planning process. It provides the final link in the circle of care planning, bringing you back to assessing the needs of your patients once again.

Appendix A
Suzy Clarke

Scenario

Suzy Clarke is a 20-year-old student nurse of 16 months. She moved away from home (100 miles away) to start her nursing programme. She gets on well with her family and has a very close relationship with all of them, dad, mum and three sisters, but due to finances she only sees them when on holiday and phones once a week. She states that she feels 'unsafe and lonely' as a consequence of this lack of contact. At first Suzy lived in university accommodation, but recently (four months ago) she moved into private rented accommodation with two friends from university. The house is small and in a 'rundown area' and, although she has her own room, all other facilities are shared. Like Suzy, one of the friends, Claire, is tidy and willing to help in the house. The other friend, Louise, is apt to forget to wash the dishes, clean the bath, use her own food, abide by the rules about heating, telephone use, etc. This causes tension between the three friends, although Claire usually takes the line of least resistance and makes excuses for Louise. This frustrates Suzy very much, which adds to the tension, and arguments often ensue; although she doesn't like the arguing, Suzy states that 'at least it relieves the tension'. Now it is winter, the house is cold and damp, there are several outstanding repairs that need attention and, despite frequent requests to the landlord, nothing is ever done. He always responds by saying that he is 'going to fix it'; all this does is anger and frustrate Suzy.

Suzy likes clubbing and house parties and normally mixes well with her peers. As with most students, money is in short supply and Suzy finds she is always overdrawn at the bank; this situation has got worse since the move to the flat, because she doesn't know how to budget her money. The first things she cuts back on are food and heating costs. She has recently lost weight 6.3 kg (1 stone); she is 1.7 m (5'7") and now 50.8 kg (8 stone). Her diet is high in simple carbohydrates and sugar and low in protein, fresh fruit and vegetables, which are seen as 'too expensive'. She tends to eat sandwiches at university and snacks on biscuits, chips and pot noodles at home; she drinks a lot of cola, approximately three litres per day. At present she is constipated and only manages to pass a small amount of hard, dark stool every three days (there is no blood, pain or mucus present). Her normal pattern is to pass a soft, formed stool every day, although she isn't doing anything about the constipation. She is spending more money on cigarettes; she used to smoke the occasional cigarette at parties, but the last three months she has taken to smoking 10–15 per day. She is reluctant to cut down as she sees this as her only pleasure and way of devoting time to herself.

Suzy has noticed a difference since she started smoking; she has a non-productive cough in the morning and gets out of breath when she runs (more than 100 yards) or climbs a flight of stairs. She has had 6 colds in the past 10 months and at present her throat is red and inflamed. Her alcohol intake has also increased since she moved into the flat, from 10 units over seven days to 32 units per week – mostly at weekends when there are house parties and trips to night clubs with her friends. She doesn't think she is drinking too much.

She is confident that she has chosen the right career, and enjoys both the practice and theory experiences, but recently she has found it difficult to keep up with the work. She has 'forgotten' to write her personal/professional journal on a regular basis and now the hand-in date is looming for her assignment and the exam is very near. Suzy has decided to concentrate on her forthcoming exam, but there always seems to be 'something else to do'. She has left the revision until a week before the exam, telling herself that she can 'cram', a technique she has had moderate success with in the past, although she didn't have other commitments at that time. However the 'cramming' doesn't appear to be effective because of the 'other things that need doing'; she is revising from 10 p.m. to 2 a.m. every night. The 'other things' don't seem to get done either because she is so tired and usually ends up falling asleep on her bed for a few hours during the day and early evening. When she finally goes to bed she cannot settle until 3 a.m. and sleeps 'fitfully' until 7 a.m., a pattern very different to her normal 11 p.m. to 7 a.m. undisturbed sleep. She is having to take 'naps in the day' to cope and as a consequence sometimes misses classes at university. Every morning she feels 'exhausted'. Suzy's relationship with her boyfriend is also strained. They tend to argue a lot and at times Suzy suggests that 'Matt is useless and unorganised; he really cannot see the wood for the trees' – comments that really could be used to describe Suzy. She does acknowledge that, at times, she thinks that the arguing is because of the stressors rather than Matt's faults. Despite this Matt still rings her regularly and desperately wants to 'sort things out' and make a go of it.

Six weeks ago Suzy was watching television (she had planned to do some work on her assignment and couldn't get this out of her mind), when she experienced a panic attack. She experienced an 'overwhelming sense of impending doom' and felt as if she was 'going to suffocate'. Her immediate thought was that she 'would die'. She had palpitations, tightness in her chest, sweaty palms, and tingling lips and fingers. She was admitted to A&E, seen by a doctor and discharged later that evening with a diagnosis of 'panic attack'.

Since that night Suzy has had six further episodes of panic for 'no apparent reason' and is now very frightened of repeat episodes. She is convinced that there is something seriously wrong with her and that the doctors are missing the signs, so much so that she has seen her GP ten times in four weeks. During the consultations Suzy has explained to her doctor that she is normally a 'coper', that she 'has never been like this before; tired, with constant colds and sore throats'. Suzy has tried to convince her GP that the attacks are a sign that there is something seriously wrong with her 'like my heart or a brain tumour'. At college she had lots of energy to play hockey and netball; she had a good appetite and never had symptoms like tiredness, headaches, constipation and feeling run down. Now she is having frequent headaches, about five times a week; she describes them as 'tight and throbbing', but says that there are no visual disturbances. She comments that she feels dizzy when she stands up from a sitting or lying position and feels like 'she is going to die'. Finally the GP offers her a full health check:

> *BLOOD RESULTS: Hb 10.8 g/dL (below normal), full blood count normal but ESR slightly raised, biochemical profile normal (12.10.12). GP prescribed iron and vitamin supplement from 17.10.12.*

VITAL SIGNS: BP 110/6 sitting and at rest, 100/60 on standing, pulse 96, strong and regular, temp 37.5. Respirations 20, rapid and shallow.

CHEST X-RAY: No abnormalities detected.

HEART AND LUNGS: No abnormalities detected.

MENSTRUATION: Normally every 28 days for 5 days moderate to light flow, now irregular, light flow, uses oral contraception but sometimes forgets to take the tablets.

URINALYSIS: No abnormalities detected.

This week Suzy has come to the GP complaining of vaginal redness, itching and discharge, with a burning pain when passing urine. Her menstrual cycle this month is regular, with a normal flow for her and she has not had a change in sexual partner. Results from high vaginal swab (13.10.12) indicates *Candida albicans* (thrush), oral medication prescribed by GP today on 17.10.12.

Imagine you are Suzy's practice nurse; the GP has sent Suzy to you to help her with her problems. Using Roper, Logan and Tierney's model, devise a plan of care with Suzy.

Assessment

Maintaining a safe environment

Previous home environment 'very comfortable and safe', present house – small, cold/damp in bedrooms in a 'rundown area', own room but all other facilities are shared. Despite frequent requests to landlord there are several serious outstanding repairs, this angers and frustrates Suzy – feels unsafe and lonely. Always had financial support from mum and dad, now overdrawn at bank. Lacks ability to devise a budget, ignoring bank statements. Never had anaemia before – Hb 10.8 g/dL, full blood count normal, raised ESR biochemical profile normal (13.10.12.). Diet lacking in iron, vitamins and minerals. Has frequent headaches (tight, throbbing, five per week, no visual disturbances, on scale of 1–10 is 9 at worst and 4 at best), dizzy on standing from lying/sitting. Thinks GP is 'missing something'. GP has diagnosed anaemia, prescribed iron tablets and vitamin supplement for 12 weeks.

Communicating

Moved away from home (100 miles) to start nursing programme, 16 months ago. Very close relationship with dad, mum and three sisters, but due to finances only sees them on holiday/phones once a week. Strained relationships with flatmates about sharing of household tasks and house rules. Misses family a lot, arguing/anger seen as way of coping with flatmates and general stressors. Has not contacted the university support services or academic supervisor.

Breathing

Used to smoke occasional cigarette, increased to 10–15 per day, over last three months. House – damp and cold, developed non-productive cough in mornings, gets out of breath (when runs more than 100 yards or climbs a flight of stairs). Had 6 colds in past 10 months, throat now red and inflamed over past four days. Vital signs: BP 110/65mmHg Hg at rest, pulse 96 bpm, strong and regular, respirations 20 breaths per minute, rapid and shallow. Reluctant to cut down smoking as sees it as her only pleasure/way of devoting time to herself. Chest X-ray, examination of heart and lungs: no abnormalities detected by GP.

Eating and drinking

Mum made sure had 'well-balanced diet' at home, now eats diet high in simple carbohydrates, sugar, and low in protein, fresh fruit and veg. Drinks approx three litres of cola per day. Does understand what a healthy diet is but cuts back on food/heating due to finances. Lost weight 6.3 kg (1 stone in six weeks); she is 1.7 m (5'7") and now 50.8 kg (8 stone).

Eliminating

Usual bowel habit – soft, formed stool every day, now constipated – passing 'small amount of hard, dark stool every three days (no blood, pain or mucus). Eats poor diet. Not taking any action to remedy constipation – GP prescribed osmotic laxative on 17.10.12. Usually no problems passing urine, urinalysis: no abnormalities detected, has a burning, stinging pain when passing urine – past 2 days – pain score 8 at worst, 5 at best on scale of 1–10, feels miserable. GP has diagnosed *Candida albicans*.

Personal cleansing and dressing

Never had thrush before, complaining of vaginal redness, itching, white discharge, burning pain when passing urine, no change in sexual partner. Wears tight jeans most of time, uses soap products to wash vaginal area, diet high in sugar, uses oral contraception, has unprotected sex with partner – feels 'unclean and dirty'. High vaginal swab – *Candida albicans* (thrush) – GP prescribed oral medication.

Controlling body temperature

Family home – warm and dry, now bedrooms damp and cold in flat, landlord unhelpful in dealing with the repairs, this angers and frustrates Suzy. Cuts back on heating the flat because of finances. Temp 37.5, throat is sore, red and inflamed, GP diagnosed virus, not taking any medication.

Mobilising

Usually has lots of energy, plays sports; has a good appetite and never had symptoms of tiredness, headaches, constipation and feeling run down. Now gets breathless (when runs more than 100 yards or climbs a flight of stairs). Still smoking 10–15 cigarettes per day and is anaemic, Hb is 10.8 g/dL. Is anxious about the changes in her health. GP diagnosed anaemia, prescribed iron tablets and vitamin supplement for 12 weeks.

Working and playing

Likes clubbing and house parties, normally mixes well with peers, now tending to argue frequently with flatmates due to differing views about house rules. Relationship with boyfriend also strained, he wants to 'sort things out' and 'make a go of it'. She thinks the arguing is because of the general stressors and not because of him but ignores his calls. Alcohol intake is normally 10 units over 7 days, now 32 units per week, mostly at weekends, increased since she moved into flat. Doesn't think she is drinking too much. Confident has chosen right career, enjoys practice and theory experiences, recently finds it difficult to keep up with work – fallen behind. Is using inappropriate study techniques such as cramming and ignoring the situation, not been in contact with academic or personal supervisor at university.

Expressing sexuality

Menstruation normally 28 days/5 days, moderate to light flow. Uses oral contraception. Now irregular, light flow, sometimes forgets to take contraceptive pill. Usually has good relationship with boyfriend, but now strained; argue all of the time. Can see that she sometimes blames boyfriend for her faults and problems. Despite this, boyfriend wants to 'sort things out' and make a go of it.

Sleeping

Normal pattern of sleep 11 p.m.–7 a.m., undisturbed, now revising 10 p.m.–2 a.m. every night, cannot settle when goes to bed until 3 a.m., then sleeps 'fitfully' until 7 a.m. Feels 'exhausted'. Not coping with assessment demands of nursing programme, feels stressed. Naps for 2–3 hours in daytime – sometimes misses classes at university, not contacted academic or personal supervisor.

Dying

States has always been a 'coper', but not coping at the moment – seen GP ten times in four weeks. States 'never been like this, tired, with constant colds and sore throats'. Six weeks ago experienced 'overwhelming sense of impending doom', felt as if she was 'going to suffocate', and thought she 'would die'. Palpitations, tightness in chest, sweaty palms, tingling lips and fingers. Admitted to A&E – discharged later that evening – diagnosis 'panic attack'. Has had six further episodes of panic – 'no apparent reason', now very frightened of repeat episodes. Panic rating – 9 at worst and 5 at best, using scale of 1–10. Is very stressed, has high caffeine intake/ (three litres of cola and six coffees per day). Convinced there is something seriously wrong – heart problems or brain tumour – that doctors are missing the signs. Full health check given by GP – no abnormalities detected in lungs or heart.

Care plan — 17 October 2012

No.	Problem	Goal	Nursing Intervention
1.	**Actual problem** Suzy says she is frightened of dying because of the 'panic attacks' that she is experiencing **Baselines** + 6 attacks in 6 weeks + Tightness in chest + Sweating + Tingling lips and fingers + Palpitations + Panic rating – 9 at worst, 5 at best using scale 1–10 + 'Overwhelming sense of doom' + 'Sure that there is something seriously wrong'	Short term: + Suzy will be able to control her feelings of panic to an acceptable level of 2 by 31.10.12 Long term: + Suzy will not experience 'panic attacks' by 19.12.12	(a) Registered nurse to discuss the anatomy and physiology of panic attacks with Suzy, making use of her existing knowledge base on 17.10.12 and answer any questions she may have at each visit (b) Registered nurse to teach Suzy breathing and relaxation exercises to help deal with the 'panic attacks' when they occur on 17.10.12, discuss her ability to use these strategies at each visit and record (*Recheck and ongoing evaluation*) (c) Suzy to practise breathing and relaxation exercises on a daily basis and use when the 'panic attacks' occur (d) Suzy to attend stress management sessions on Mon evenings as from 22.10.12 (e) Registered nurse to explain the principles of classical conditioning to Suzy and how the above strategies will help her deal with her experience on 17.10.12 and answer any questions at each visit (f) Registered nurse to evaluate the effectiveness of breathing/relaxation and stress management sessions using recheck information, baselines and goals on 31.10.12 and 19.12.12 and record (*Final evaluation*)

No.	Problem	Goal	Nursing Intervention
2.	**Actual problem** Suzy feels she is 'not coping' and feels 'unsafe' due to the recent life changes **Baselines** + Lacks study skills – time management – fallen behind with assignment/exam revision + Lacks financial management skills – overdrawn at the bank + Has accommodation problems – house damp, cold, outstanding repairs + Arguing with flatmates about household tasks and living together + Coping scale of 1–10; 8 at worst and 2 at best	Short term: + Suzy will have arranged appointments with her academic supervisor, personal banker and student services by 20.10.12 + Suzy will rate her feelings of 'not being able to cope' at the level of 2 by 14.11.12 Long term: + Suzy will feel in control of the factors that are causing her to feel that she is 'not coping' and 'unsafe' by 19.12.12	(a) Registered nurse to discuss situation with Suzy and agree an action plan on 17.10.12 that involves Suzy making an appointment with her academic supervisor, personal banker, student services and academic supervisor (b) Suzy to arrange a house meeting with her flatmates to devise a set of house rules and cleaning rota on 17.10.12 (c) Registered nurse to discuss effectiveness of 2(a,b) with Suzy discuss at each visit and record (*Recheck and ongoing evaluation*) (d) Registered nurse to discuss the effectiveness of 2(a,b) with Suzy using the recheck information, baselines and goals on 20.10.12, 14.11.12 and 19.12.08 and record (*Final evaluation*)

No.	Problem	Goal	Nursing Intervention
3.	**Actual problem** Suzy says she is 'not eating a well-balanced diet due to lack of money and motivation. She has lost weight and is having problems opening her bowels.' **Baselines** ✦ Bowels open every 3 days, hard, dark stools, no blood or mucus ✦ Does understand what a healthy diet consists of ✦ Diet is high in sugar, low in protein, fruit and veg, mainly processed food ✦ Has a limited budget and lacks motivation to shop and prepare food ✦ Weight 50.8 kg (8 stone), height 1.7m (5'7")	Short term: ✦ Suzy will plan a menu plan and allocate a budget for food by 24.10.12 ✦ Suzy will eat a diet that is high in complex carbohydrates, protein, fruit and veg, low in fat, low cost by 24.10.12 ✦ Suzy will open her bowels once daily by 24.10.12 Long term: ✦ Suzy will weigh 8 stones 7 lb by 19.12.12	(a) Registered nurse to discuss with Suzy the requirements of an affordable, healthy, well-balanced diet on 17.10.12 and answer any questions at each visit (b) Suzy to devise a menu and food budget plan that allows her to adapt her dietary and fluid intake on 18.10.12 (c) Suzy to attend well-person clinic at 2-weekly intervals for support and weight check as from 17.10.12 (d) Suzy to take osmotic laxative as prescribed by her GP (e) Registered nurse to discuss the effectiveness of the above interventions at each appointment and record (*Recheck and ongoing evaluation*) (f) Registered nurse to evaluate the effectiveness of the above interventions using recheck information, baselines and goals on 24.10.12 and 19.12.12 and record (*Final evaluation*)

No.	Problem	Goal	Nursing Intervention
4.	**Actual problem** Suzy says she has pain when 'passing urine', due to thrush **Baselines** ✦ Pain is 6 on scale of 1–10, 'burns and stings' when passing urine, feels miserable ✦ Vaginal redness, white discharge, yeasty odour ✦ Itching at worst 8 and at best 5 on comfort scale of 1–10 ✦ High vaginal swab – results on 17.10.12 positive to *Candida albicans*	Short term: ✦ Suzy will be able to pass urine without pain by 20.10.12 ✦ Suzy will have a comfort level of 2 or less by 20.10.12 ✦ Results from high vaginal swab will be negative to *Candida albicans* by 31.10.12	(a) Registered nurse to discuss the possible causes of 'thrush' with Suzy and help identify the triggering factors on 17.10.12 (b) Registered nurse to explain the action and side effects of the medication to Suzy and answer any questions on 17.10.12 (c) Suzy to take the prescribed medication for her thrush on 17.10.12 (d) Registered nurse to discuss with Suzy ways to ease the discomfort she feels as a result of the thrush on 17.10.12 (e) Suzy to return for high vaginal swab on 29.10.12 (*Recheck*) (f) Registered nurse to evaluate effectiveness of the above interventions using the baselines and goals on 20.10.12 and 31.10.12 and record (*Final evaluation*)
5.	**Actual problem** Suzy says she is 'exhausted', has frequent headaches and feels dizzy when standing from a sitting position due to anaemia **Baselines** ✦ Hb 10.8 g/dL on 17.10.08 ✦ Headaches (5 per week, no visual disturbances). On a scale of 1–10; 9 at worst and 4 at best, tight, throbbing pain ✦ BP standing 100/60mmHg – sitting at rest 110/65	Long term: ✦ Suzy's haemoglobin level will be within limits of 12–14 by 16.1.13 ✦ Suzy's headaches will cease by 28.11.12 ✦ Suzy will not feel dizzy when standing from a sitting position by 16.1.13	(a) Suzy to eat foods that are high in iron and vitamin C when possible (b) Suzy to take iron and vitamin supplement as prescribed by the GP for 12 weeks from 17.10.12 (c) Registered nurse to take blood sample (full biochemical profile and blood count) on 14.1.13 and liaise with GP following results if necessary (*Recheck*) (d) Registered nurse to discuss the effectiveness of 5(a,b) at each appointment and record (*Recheck and ongoing evaluation*) (e) Registered nurse to evaluate the effectiveness of 5 (a,b) using the baselines and goals on 16.1.13 and record (*Final evaluation*)

Evaluation of progress

Date	Care delivered (use intervention number from care plan)	Evaluation of care
17.10.2012	1(a,b,c,d); 2(a); 3(a,c), 4(a,b,c,d)	+ Can demonstrate breathing and relaxation techniques following teaching today
20.10.2012	1(a,b,c,d); 2(c,d), 3(a,d,e), 4(f), 5(a,b,d)	+ Suzy had a panic attack last night, panic rating 4, lasted 4 minutes, used breathing techniques which helped settle the panic and gave her 'some control' of the situation. Practised breathing techniques and discussed the process of classical conditioning during the visit
		+ Suzy has made appointments as per plan; will attend first appointment on 22.10.12 with academic supervisor, 23.10.12 with student services has got plan of action ready to discuss with her. Suzy discussed rota and need to identify house rules with flatmates on 17.10.12, friends seem to accept need to change, have started task. Suzy's coping level is 6 today
		+ Has completed 7 days of menu plans, meals reflect diet requirements. Bowels open today – still hard but no pain, mucus or blood. Had headache yesterday on waking, Pain score was 6, no pain today
		+ Has not yet completed budget plan, is waiting until she sees personal banker on 23.10.12
		+ No pain when passing urine since 19.10.12, comfort level now 1. Vagina still a little sore, but no discharge or odour

Appendix B
George Brown

Scenario

George Brown is 68 years old; he lives with his wife Elsie in a comfortable two-bedroom bungalow that they own. His wife, who was requesting 'nursing help', referred him to the district nursing team. The team knew George, as his GP had asked them to visit twice previously, but he declined nursing help on both occasions, saying that he did not require any care.

He has worked hard all his life as head gardener for the parks department and has enjoyed 'good health until recently'. He normally eats three meals a day and his usual sleep pattern is 10.30 p.m. to 7.00 a.m., waking twice to pass urine. He prefers to avoid his doctor's surgery and dislikes 'bothering the doctors and nurses'. George is profoundly deaf and has worn a hearing aid for 18 years; he can lip-read very well and, when his hearing aid is switched on, he achieves a good level of communication. Eight years ago George was diagnosed as having type 2 diabetes; this is controlled by diet and oral medication. Both Elsie and George understand the management of his condition very well and the need for preventative intervention. Elsie tests his urine weekly (it is usually negative for glucose and ketones) and the chiropodist visits every six weeks.

George retired to the seaside four years ago and remains very close to his son and two grandchildren who live in a city about 13 miles away. They are enjoying their retirement near the sea and their family and hobbies. His interests are gardening, dancing, crown green bowling and walking with Elsie; they own a car and used to lead a 'busy social life', meeting with friends 3–4 times a week for a coffee, lunch or an evening meal at the local pub. Now they are not going out with their friends at all and George is not engaged in any of his hobbies. The family relies on their help and advice on caring for the grandchildren and general support. Elsie manages the household finances (she always has done), and George relies upon her guidance and judgement greatly.

Four years ago, a malignant tumour was discovered in George's large bowel; he had an abdominal resection of the colon and formation of a temporary colostomy. Elsie nursed George until he returned to hospital 18 months later for reversal of his colostomy. Whilst in hospital he developed acute retention of urine. On investigation of this, a tumour of the prostate gland was found, which was removed; however, on his six-monthly check the consultant identified that the cancer had spread to his bladder and testes. Since the surgery George has frequent (6–8 daily), watery, pale yellow stools, swollen testes and penis and occasional urinary incontinence (2–3 times a week, usually at night). He states he some-times has problems 'holding his water' until he reaches the toilet. He passes urine 8–10 times daily, which is a pale yellow straw colour with no pain or odour; he states that he feels 'sore and uncomfortable' after opening his bowels; on a comfort scale of 1–10, it is at best 6 and at worst 9. He states that the pain in his testes is a constant, uncomfortable, dull ache and makes him feel irritable; on a scale of 1–10, the pain is at best 7 and at worst 10; he is not wearing underpants at present; the skin on his scrotum and penis is unbroken and pink.

Six months ago, George had an emergency operation for a perforated gastric ulcer; he made an uneventful recovery and returned home to Elsie. He is now terminally ill, experiencing a great deal of bone pain (due to the spread of cancer), especially in his ribs and lower back. Due to the previous gastric ulcer, he cannot take aspirin or anti-inflammatory drugs. His GP has prescribed morphine tablets, which George is taking every six hours as prescribed, but as an opiate they are not completely effective for bone pain. The pain is somewhat relieved by Elsie massaging the area with Deep Heat™ cream. George says the pain 'feels like toothache', makes him feel 'fed-up' and using a category scale of 1–10 (agreed with George) he rates the severity of the pain as '7 at its worst and 3 at its best'. George did smoke 20 years ago and, although he has a chronic non-productive cough, he has no breathing or circulatory problems. His complexion is pale and sallow, and there are no breaks or red areas on his skin. He has no history of anaemia and his blood test results are within normal limits (12.11.12). Respirations 14 breaths per minute, no difficulty breathing, pulse 90 beats per minute, good volume and rhythmic, blood pressure 140/90mmHg. On testing the urine (19.11.12) nothing abnormal was detected; it was pale yellow straw-coloured with no odour or pain on passing. He has been offered laundry and continence services but has refused at present. He has always had a good appetite and usually weighs 76.2 kg (12 stone); he is 1.78 m (5 feet 10 inches). He has lost 15.88 kg (2.5 stones) in the past six months; however, he tolerates small amounts of food at each mealtime, but sometimes misses meals due to the pain.

George's mobility has severely declined in the past three weeks and he can now only manage to walk around the house. His gait has become very unsteady even with the use of a stick; there are a coal fire, three pets and many loose rugs in the home for George to negotiate. His normal sleep pattern is disturbed: usually no more than two hours a night and very restless, sometimes sleeping in a chair because of the lower back and rib pain. He has become reluctant to use his hearing aid, does not look forward to his family visiting and finds he does not want to mix with his friends. He states he is 'fed-up and tired', using a category scale of 1–10 (agreed with George), 9 at worst and 3 at best, choosing to turn off his hear-ing aid as a means of escape. George appears to be unaware of his diagnosis and prognosis, but Elsie is fully aware of both. She expresses a strong need to care for George, which she manages in a loving and successful manner. However, just lately she has found that 'things are getting her down'; she misses the interaction with their friends, but is reluctant to leave George unattended. Despite George's reluctant attitude, she feels that she would like help from the nursing team.

Assessment (nursing history): date completed 19.11.12

The information from the nursing history is categorised under the universal self-care requisites, but health deviation self-care requisites and developmental self-care requisites are also considered.

Sufficient intake of air

George did smoke 20 years ago (20 per day for 40 years) and, although he has a chronic non-productive cough, he has no breathing or circulatory problems. Respiration rate 14 per minute, regular, Blood pressure 140/90mmHg, pulse 90 beats per minute, good volume and rhythm. He has a pale/sallow complexion but his mucous membranes are pink. No history of anaemia, blood test results are within normal limits, haemoglobin 11.8 g/100 millilitres (12.11.12).

Sufficient intake of water and food

George has type 2 diabetes diagnosed in 2004, controlled by diet and oral medication; both Elsie and George understand the management of his condition very well. Despite history of gastric ulcer, normally has a good appetite (three meals a day), but recently (within past six months) has lost weight 15.88 kg (2.5 stones), usually 76.2 kg (12 stone), 1.78 m (5 feet 10"), now only manages small amounts of food at each meal, sometimes misses meals, due to pain. Due to previous gastric ulcer, cannot take aspirin or anti-inflammatory drugs to control pain in ribs and lower back.

Satisfactory eliminative functions

Due to past surgery has 'frequent loose stools' (6–8 daily), watery, pale yellow, no blood or pain. Due to the spread of prostate cancer he has swollen testes and penis and occasional urinary incontinence 2–3 times a week, usually at night. He states that the pain in his testes is a constant, uncomfortable, dull ache and makes him feel irritable; on a scale of 1–10, the pain is at best 7 and at worst 10; he is not wearing underpants at present. The skin on the scrotum and penis is intact and pink. George says that he feels 'sore and uncomfortable' after opening his bowels; on a comfort scale of 1–10, it is 6 at best and 9 at worst. He states he sometimes has problems 'holding his water' until he reaches the toilet. Passes urine 8–10 times daily that is a pale yellow/straw colour, with no pain or odour. Due to the occasional urinary incontinence he has requested a urinal to avoid getting up to the toilet at night. They have declined laundry and continence services at present. Elsie tests urine weekly and records, normally negative to glucose and ketones. Tested on 19.11.12, no abnormalities detected.

Activity balanced with rest

Was a head gardener for the parks dept, enjoyed 'good health until recently'. George's gait is unsteady even with use of stick, his mobility has severely declined in the past three weeks, previously George enjoyed gardening, dancing, bowls and walking with Elsie, now can only manage to walk around the house, due to generalised weakness. Sleep pattern is normally 10.30 p.m. to 7.00 a.m. but now has a restless sleep (no more than two hours), sometimes sleeping in a chair due to unrelieved pain in ribs and lower back.

Balance between solitude and social interaction

Retired to the seaside town four years ago, after very much looking forward to retirement from his job as head gardener to the parks department. He has one son and two grandsons who live in a city about 13 miles away. George and Elsie say they are very close to their family, and used to lead a busy social life, meeting with friends 3-4 times a week for a coffee, lunch or an evening meal at the local pub. Now they are not going out with their friends at all. George usually uses his hearing aid to achieve good levels of communication and can lip-read very well. Is profoundly deaf and has become reluctant to use his hearing aid (past three months); he is finding he doesn't want to mix with his friends and doesn't look forward to his family visiting. Elsie says 'I really miss seeing our friends but I don't feel I can leave George on his own.' George says 'I am fed-up and tired.' George often chooses to turn off his hearing aid when friends and family visit. Elsie manages the home and the finances (she always has done). George relies upon her support, guidance and judgement greatly.

Prevention of hazards to human life, human functioning and human well-being

There is a coal fire, many loose mats and three pets, and both George and Elsie are aware of George's unsteady gait; a fireguard and smoke detectors are in place. Both are aware of the preventative intervention needed for the management of diabetes; a chiropodist visits every six weeks. George has a lot of pain in his ribs and lower back which is relieved by Elsie massaging with 'Deep Heat™ cream', 'feels like constant toothache', makes him feel fed-up, using category scale of 1–10 (agreed with George) rates pain as '7 worst and 3 best'. Currently taking prescribed morphine tablets six-hourly, but are not very effective. There are no breaks or red areas on George's skin, but due to incontinence, frequent loose stools, and immobility, may be at risk of developing pressure sores. Doesn't have any aids or adaptations to alleviate pressure on sitting/lying at present.

Promotion of human functioning and development within social groups in accordance with human potential, known human limitations and the desire for 'normalcy'

George has coped with his deafness and diabetes very successfully for many years. He feels that since his operations he can normally cope with his frequent bowel movements, occasional incontinence and swollen testes, but finds over the last few weeks his tolerance to these problems is weakened by the constant pain. It is also isolating him from his family, friends and recreation, and affects his sleep and activities, George admits he uses deafness and switching off his hearing aid as a means of escape. He states he is 'fed-up and tired', using a category scale of 1–10 (agreed with George), 9 at worst and 3 at best. GP suggested nursing help on several occasions but George declined, 'prefers to manage himself,' 'dislikes bothering nurses and doctors'. Elsie would now like some 'nursing help' as 'things are getting her down'. George and Elsie have worked hard all their lives and were enjoying their retirement near the sea and their hobbies and family. Their family relies on their help and advice with caring for their children and general issues. George wants to regain his former independence for as long as he possibly can.

Identified healthcare deficits

1. Pain
2. Swollen testes and penis
3. Urinary incontinence
4. Frequency of bowel movements
5. Feelings of isolation and being 'fed-up'
6. Potential deficit – pressure ulcers on sacrum and scrotum

Care plan — 19 November 2012

No.	Problem/Need statement	Goals (prescriptive operations)	Implementation (treatment operations)
1.	George states 'I have pain in my ribs and lower back'	**Short term:**	(a) Elsie and nurse to encourage George to take prescribed tablets at 08:00, 14:00, 20:00, 02:00 (if awake)
		+ George will state that his pain level is 3 or less by 26.11.12	(b) Elsie to apply Deep Heat™ cream every 6 hours to George's lower back and ribs
	Baselines	+ George will state that he is less fed-up, with a score of below 3 by 26.11.12	(c) George to assess his pain using the pain scale in between the medication regime at 10:00, 16:00, 22:00 and record on the pain chart (*Recheck and ongoing evaluation*)
	+ Constant	+ George will sleep for 4 hours undisturbed by 26.11.12	(d) Nurse to assess pain levels by asking George and record responses on the pain chart at each visit (*Recheck and ongoing evaluation*)
	+ Feels like toothache		
	+ Feels 'fed-up' category scale 1–10, worst 9 best 3	**Long term:**	(e) George to record quality and quantity of sleep and how he feels each morning (*Recheck*)
	+ Pain category scale 1–10, worst 7, best 3	+ George will state that he is pain-free at all times by 17.12.12	(f) Nurse/Elsie to liaise with GP if George feels pain medication is not effective in controlling pain
	+ Sleeps 2 hours of very restless sleep per night, in chair		(g) Nurse to evaluate care on 26.11.12 and 17.12.12 using baselines and goals and record (*Final evaluation*)
2.	George states that he has 'frequent loose stools' due to previous bowel surgery; he says 'I feel sore and uncomfortable'	**Short term:**	(a) Elsie to record when George has bowels open, nurse to assess using baseline and record at each visit (*Recheck and ongoing evaluation*)
		+ George will state that his comfort score is 6 or less by 23.11.12	(b) George to be encouraged to drink at least one litre of fluids per day, ensuring no artificial sweeteners present and eat low-residue diet
	Baselines		(c) George/Elsie to apply prescribed barrier cream to sore areas after George has had his bowels opened and assess and record condition of the skin, report to nurse if condition deteriorates
	+ Passes stools 6–8 times daily, watery, pale yellow, no pain, no blood		

No.	Problem/Need statement	Goals (prescriptive operations)	Implementation (treatment operations)
	+ Area surrounding anus red, dry, but skin unbroken + Doesn't feel able to cope any more and states 'it is getting me down' + Comfort scale 1–10, worst 9, best 6	+ The area surrounding the anus will be free from redness and hydrated by 23.11.12 + George will state that he can cope with the 'frequent bowel movements' by 26.11.12	(d) Nurse to discuss with George and Elsie their ability to cope with George's hygiene requirements and frequency of bowel movements at each visit and record (*Recheck and ongoing evaluation*) (e) Nurse to evaluate using goals and baselines on 23.11.12 and 26.11.12 and record (*Final evaluation*)
3.	George says he has occasional problems 'holding his water' until he can reach the toilet due to tiredness **Baselines** + No abnormalities detected on testing – 19.11.12 + 8–10 times daily, pale yellow/straw, no odour or pain + Incontinent 2–3 times a week, usually at night	Short term: + George will be able to 'pass water' when necessary and in an appropriate place by 23.11.12	(a) Elsie to record when and where George passes urine (*Recheck*) (b) Nurse to assess George's ability to pass urine as needed, using baseline at each visit and record (*Recheck and ongoing evaluation*) (c) Nurse to liaise with GP if there is a deviation from the baseline or any further problems are expressed (d) Nurse to supply urinal and continence pads for use at night, on 20.11.12, and their effectiveness with George at each visit and record (*Recheck and ongoing evaluation*) (e) Nurse to evaluate using baselines and goals on 23.11.12 and record (*Final evaluation*)

No.	Problem/Need statement	Goals (prescriptive operations)	Implementation (treatment operations)
4.	George feels 'uncomfortable and irritable' due to swollen testes and penis **Baselines** + Pain – constant, uncomfortable, dull ache makes him feel irritable; scale of 1–10, worst 10 best 7 + Skin on scrotum and penis is pink, intact with no blemishes or breaks	Short term: + George will state his pain level is 7 or less by 26.11.12 Long term: + The skin on George's scrotum and penis will remain free from redness and intact at all times	(a) Nurse to discuss with George and Elsie the swelling, condition of skin on scrotum and penis, pain and comfort level at each visit and record (*Recheck and ongoing evaluation*) (b) Nurse/Elsie to encourage George to wear scrotal support or two pairs of underpants at all times (c) Nurse to liaise with GP if there is a deviation from the baseline or any further problems are expressed (d) Nurse to evaluate using baselines and goals on 26.11.12 and record (*Final evaluation*)
5.	George states that he feels 'fed-up and isolated' because of his recent illness, pain and incontinence **Baselines** + Turning hearing aid off when friends and family visit + 'I don't feel like mixing with anyone right now' + Fed-up scale 0–10, 9 worst, 2 best	Short term: + George will state that his feelings of being 'isolated and fed-up' will be 2 or less by 26.11.12 + George will meet with his friends and family with his hearing aid switched on by 26.11.12 Long term: + George will be free from the factors that make him feel isolated and rejoin the social activities of his choosing by 19.12.12	(a) Nurse/Elsie to check hearing aid is switched on, speak slowly and clearly facing George during all communications/interactions (b) Nurse to offer reassurance, explanations and advice to Elsie and George, where appropriate, to alleviate anxious feelings or worries (c) George/Elsie to attend Age Concern luncheon club on Wednesdays and Fridays; nurse to arrange sitter when George cannot attend (d) Nurse to discuss the effectiveness of 5(a,b,c) at each visit using baselines and record (*Recheck and ongoing evaluation*) (e) Nurse to evaluate using goals and baseline on 26.11.12 and 19.12.12 and record (*Final evaluation*)

No.	Problem/Need statement	Goals (prescriptive operations)	Implementation (treatment operations)
6.	Due to recent weight loss, immobility and incontinence George is at risk of developing pressure ulcers **Baseline** ✚ All areas prone to pressure are intact and free from redness	✚ George's skin will remain intact and free from redness at all times	(a) Elsie to observe all areas at risk of developing pressure ulcers during care provision and report to nurse any signs of redness, dryness or breaks to the skin *(Recheck)* (b) Nurse to liaise with George and Elsie and assess the condition of George's skin using the baseline and record at every visit *(Recheck and ongoing evaluation)* (c) Nurse/Elsie to encourage George to be mobile within his own limits every hour during the day (when awake) (d) George to use special cushions/mattress at all times (e) Elsie to apply prescribed cream to any red/sore unbroken areas on skin as needed (f) Nurse to evaluate using baselines and goals at each visit and record *(Final evaluation)*

Evaluation of progress

Date	Care delivered (use intervention number from care plan)	Evaluation of care
20.11.2012	1(abcde), 2(abcd), 3(abd), 4(ab), 5(abd), 6(abcdf)	+ Pain score 6 at 14:00 hrs – pain remains as baseline. George and Elsie reassured that new pain medication will take another 24 hours to become established + Urinal and continence pads supplied to George + Elsie states 'George is still not switching on his hearing aid, we don't seem to have moved forward very much.' Fed-up scale unchanged from baseline. Reassured that the new care measures will take 24–48 hours to start taking effect + George is using the pressure-relieving equipment, pressure areas – no redness and skin intact
21.11.12	1(abcde), 2(abcd), 3(abd), 4(ab), 5(abcd), 6(abcdf)	+ Over past 24 hours pain score has ranged from 3 to 5, now 4 at 14:30 hrs. George states, 'I slept for 3 hours without waking last night and I think I feel a little better, things are improving' + Scrotal support provided too small, changed for larger size. George is wearing new style of underpants bought by Elsie and he is a little more comfortable: 8 at worst and 5 at best + Elsie has enjoyed luncheon club today: 'I felt as though I could relax for the first time for weeks, knowing that someone was looking after George for me.' George slept whilst the sitter was there. He has not communicated with his friends or family today. Fed-up score 8
22.11.12	1(abcde), 2(abcd), 3(add), 4(ab), 5(abd), 6(abcdf)	+ George switched on his hearing aid during a visit from his son

Date	Care delivered (use intervention number from care plan)	Evaluation of care
23.11.12	1(abcde), 2(abcde), 3(abde), 4(ab), 5(abcd), 6(abcdf)	+ Comfort score 6. Skin around anus is pink, but supple, no signs of breaks. George states 'I am coping much better, it's not as sore now.' Is managing to drink 1250 ml fluid a day and small amounts at meal times, with a few snacks due to being able to use the urinal at night, has not been incontinent of urine. George states 'I think that the worry of wetting myself was making it harder for me to sleep properly; now that I have the bottle, I know I don't have to drag myself to the toilet. It's given me peace of mind' + Elsie enjoyed luncheon club. George had a chat with the sitter with his hearing aid switched on, he said it was good to talk to someone distanced from his situation. Fed-up score 5
24.11.12	1(abcde), 2(abcd), 3(abd), 4(ab), 5(abd), 6(abcdf)	+ George had his hearing aid switched on during a visit from a friend
25.11.12	1(abcde), 2(abcd), 3(abd), 4(ab), 5(abd), 6(abcdf)	+ George had his hearing aid switched on during visits from his son and grandchildren. He played cards with his grandchildren for 30 minutes, which Elsie was very pleased about
26.11.12	1(abcdef), 2(abcde), 3(abd), 4(ab), 5(abde), 6(abcdf)	+ Pain level is mostly 3 by day and night, remains constant and like toothache. 3–4 hours unbroken sleep for past 2 nights. George states 'the pain is more bearable and I do feel a lot better for sleeping more' + Skin around anus is free from redness and breaks and is supple and hydrated. Comfort score 3. States 'I am feeling much better able to cope, I think part of it is that I am not feeling so tired' + The skin on scrotum remains pink and free from breaks. Pain is 6 or less, most of the time. George states 'It is less uncomfortable, now that it is supported' + George has his hearing aid switched on for most of the day and is meeting with and talking to his friends and family. He states 'I am less fed-up with myself, about a 3, I feel more sociable now that I feel more comfortable and less tired'

Appendix C
Shoaib Hameed

Scenario

Shoaib Hameed is 58 years old and is a manager for a computer software company. He is extremely good at his job, and has made great progress in the past five years by climbing the 'corporate ladder' at a rapid speed. He was a gifted student with ability for creative, original thought. He has a strong work ethic of 'you have to work hard to be successful' and quickly realised that the only way to get promotion was to go on to an intensive management programme. His job is very stressful in terms of meeting deadlines, problem solving and decision making.

He works long hours and frequently takes work home to complete or 'think about', even at the weekends. As a consequence of his work commitments he doesn't find the time to socialise and unwind. The demands on his time also prevent him from maintaining contact with his friends and even his teenage children. He says that he has no time for keeping in contact with friends, but recognises that this is making him feel isolated – a feeling that he also experiences at work as a consequence of being 'management'. He has a good relationship with his wife, Najeema, although she tends to 'nag' out of concern about his lifestyle. He tends to argue with the children even when something is not really their fault. Najeema has started visiting friends on her own and pursuing hobbies as she cannot rely on Shoaib to accompany her. She often goes to bed several hours before him because he is finishing his work. Shoaib sleeps four hours per night, partly because he goes to bed late but also because he wakes early with 'things running through his head'. They have a comfortable lifestyle, but unfortunately very little time to enjoy the rewards that his hard work brings. There is a large house to maintain with an accompanying mortgage.

There is little time for exercise and lately he has been experiencing repeated shoulder pain, especially when he has done DIY at the weekend. His GP has prescribed an anti-inflammatory drug (ibuprofen) but didn't do any further investigations.

He has tried to give up smoking three times in the past year but has found that the amount he smokes has increased to 30 per day as he uses it to deal with the stress that he feels. For religious reasons, Shoaib does not drink alcohol. His diet is generally high in fat. He does not eat pork and will only eat meat that is halal.

When he was younger, he and his wife had made plans to retire at 55 to the south of France. However, the pressures of mortgages and the introduction of university fees will mean that he will need to work until he is 70.

Earlier in the day of admission, Shoaib was carrying out some DIY when he felt a severe crushing pain in his chest and collapsed on the floor. His colour was pale grey and he was sweating profusely. His wife found him and called 999 – the paramedic crew attended quickly and took Shoaib to the local A&E. On arrival, his pulse was 120 beats per minute and BP was 90/50mmHg. An ECG indicated an acute anterior myocardial infarction (MI). Shoaib was given Diamorphine 5 mg for pain relief, and Metoclopramide 10 mg as an anti-emetic intravenously (IV). Shoaib was taken immediately to the cardiac catheter laboratory, where he underwent primary percutaneous coronary intervention (PCI) to 'open up' the blocked coronary artery that was responsible for the MI.

Following the PCI, Shoaib was transferred to the coronary care unit (CCU), where he stayed for the first part of his recovery. After admission to CCU, Shoaib has remained pain-free for 48 hours, and his condition has stabilised. MI has been confirmed through a rise in cardiac enzymes (specific substances that are usually released into the bloodstream only if the heart is damaged).

He has now been transferred to a step-down cardiology ward. Although his condition is stable, he remains very frightened. His urine output is satisfactory, but he is experiencing some problems 'going to the toilet' to have his bowels open. His wife and children have visited and appear to be very concerned about being involved in his care. Unfortunately, visiting regulations on the ward limit their visits.

Assessment summary using the Neuman Systems Model

Intrapersonal

Physical

Myocardial infarction 48 hours ago

Has been commenced on aspirin, Clopidogrel, beta-blocker, ACE inhibitor and statin

Currently pain-free – taking no analgesia

Bruising in right groin following PCI

O_2 saturation now 99% on air (norm is 95–100%)

BP 110/60mmtlg, pulse rate 75 bpm

Smokes 30 cigarettes per day

Has attempted to give up smoking 3 times in the past 12 months with no NRT

Weight 101.6 kg (16 stone), height 1.8 m (5ft 11") (BMI 32)

Doesn't drink alcohol due to religious beliefs

Has a balanced diet at home. However, diet at work is poor – usually skips lunch. Has high-fat diet when away on business

Total cholesterol 6.4 mmol/l, LDL cholesterol 4.3 mmol/l, HDL cholesterol 1 mmol/l

Has not opened bowels since admission – feels constipated and is scared of straining in case he gets more chest pain

Normally opens bowels every day

Eating small amounts, but does not like hospital food

Is wary about mobilising to the toilet due to fear of getting more chest pain, so using urine bottles most of the time

Is managing to wash most of himself with a bowl at his bed. Needs help with washing his back

Is only wearing pyjamas at present – able to dress independently

Would like to shower but is scared of suffering another MI whilst in bathroom

Has been reluctant to exercise recently due to experiencing shoulder pain on exertion

Is mobilising very gently, but is concerned about doing too much in case pain returns

Normally sleeps 4 hours per night – goes to bed late and wakes at about 5.30, worrying about work

Sleeping poorly (less than 2 hours per night) due to noise on CCU and anxiety about condition

Reluctant to have sleeping pills in case he becomes addicted

Psychosociocultural

Smokes because he feels stressed about work and money

No hearing or speech problems. Wears glasses for driving and watching TV

Stressful job – manager in IT firm. Works 12 hours a day and takes work home

Comfortable lifestyle but little time to enjoy it

Large house and mortgage

Strong work ethic

Is unhappy with size and fitness – feels that he has 'let himself go'

Developmental

Is keen to do whatever is necessary to recover from his MI, and prevent further events

Had originally planned to retire to south of France at 55 but commitments have changed these plans

Spiritual

Very anxious (anxiety level of 8 on 0–10 scale), is scared that he is going to die

Muslim faith

Feels that his Muslim faith will help him through this experience

Interpersonal

Jokes with family about being overweight

Quite withdrawn and quiet. Little interaction with healthcare team or other patients

Feels that he has little to talk about with other patients

Often feels isolated at work, and does not get enough opportunity to mix with family and friends

Has good relationship with wife and children, although it is strained by his long hours of work

Wife and children visit regularly and want to get involved in care

Shoaib feels isolated at times in hospital – 'nothing in common with other patients'

Close bond with wife

Believes that sexual relations with his wife may not be possible due to MI

Extrapersonal

Is worried about financial implications of illness

Is worried about the affects of his illness on his work colleagues

Systematic nursing diagnosis

Problem	Links to problem number
Short-term risk of further chest pain/MI	1
Risk of heart failure	1
Risk of arrhythmias	1
Risk of bleeding	1
Reduced mobility	2
Having to use urine bottles	2
Constipated	3
Difficulty sleeping	4
Anxiety about dying	5
Anxiety about future lifestyle	5
Anxiety about financial future	5
Anxiety about sex life	5
Smokes 30 per day	6
BMI is 32 – obese	6
High cholesterol	6
Medium- to long-term risk of further MI	6

Care plan problems

1	Short-term complications
2	Reduced mobility
3	Constipation
4	Difficulty sleeping
5	Anxiety regarding condition and future lifestyle
6	Rehabilitation and secondary prevention

Care plan — from 48 hours post-MI (i.e starts 22.11.12)

No.	Problem	Goal	Nursing intervention
1.	Shoaib is unaware that his condition carries the risk of complications: + further chest pain or discomfort + cardiac arrhythmias + heart failure + bleeding (due to anticoagulation following PCI) due to a lack of knowledge **Baseline** + no pain (0 on visual analogue scale), and is receiving no analgesia + currently in sinus rhythm with occasional ventricular ectopics. Heart rate is 75 bpm + Shoaib currently exhibits no symptoms of heart failure. BP 110/60mmHg, HR 75 bpm, O₂ sats 99% on air, resp rate 14/min + Shoaib currently exhibits no signs of significant bleeding. Hb 14 g/dl + Minor bruising in right groin following PCI + No knowledge of possible complications	Shoaib will be able to list the complications and identify the symptoms by 23.11.12 Shoaib will remain free of the following throughout his hospital stay: + chest pain or discomfort + cardiac arrhythmias + signs and symptoms of heart failure + bleeding	(a) Shoaib to be reminded by registered nurse caring for him on each shift to report to nursing staff: + any chest pain or discomfort + any palpitations or dizziness + any shortness of breath + any bruising, bleeding or headaches (b) Member of nursing staff to check pain levels four times daily (0800, 1200, 1600, 2200) and record (*Recheck and ongoing evaluation*) (c) Nursing staff to record BP, pulse, respiratory rate and oxygen saturations four times a day, and report any deterioration from the baselines to medical team (*Recheck and ongoing evaluation*) (d) Registered nurse to ensure that an electrocardiogram (ECG) is recorded during any pain, palpitations or dizziness, and medical staff informed of any acute changes (f) Nursing staff or cardiac technician to carry out routine ECG on 23.11.12 and on day of discharge (g) Registered nurse to inform Shoaib on 23.11.12 that risk of bleeding is increased due to the medication that he has received (h) Registered nurse to check right femoral wound site daily and report any additional bruising or swelling (*Recheck and ongoing evaluation*) (i) Registered nurse to test next bowel movement for occult blood, test urine on 23.11.12 for haematuria and report any abnormal findings to medical team (*Recheck and ongoing evaluation*) (j) Clotting screen and full blood count to be taken on 24.11.12 and 26.11.12 (k) Nurse to evaluate effectiveness of the above interventions using goals and baselines by date of discharge (*Final evaluation*)

No.	Problem / Baseline	Goal	Interventions
2.	Shoaib is concerned about 'doing too much' in case his pain returns following his recent MI **Baseline:** ✦ Shoaib is currently only mobilising gently around his bed area unassisted ✦ Confidence level is 4 at best, 2 at worst on a scale of 1–10	By the time of discharge, Shoaib will be mobilising freely and confidently around the ward Shoaib will state his confidence level is 5 or more by 23.11.12	(a) Nursing team to encourage Shoaib to mobilise gently, in line with rehabilitation programme, explaining actions to take should he experience any symptoms (b) Registered nurse caring for Shoaib on each shift to remind Shoaib to complete leg exercises every 3–4 hours (c) Nursing team to ensure that bedside environment compensates for reduced mobility (e.g. ensure urine bottles available for when Shoaib does not feel able to mobilise to toilet) (d) Registered nurse to refer Shoaib to cardiac rehabilitation team on day 3 post-MI (23.11.12) (e) Registered nurse to evaluate the effectiveness of the above interventions using goals and baselines on 23.11.12
3.	Shoaib is scared of straining when opening his bowels in case he gets chest pain **Baseline:** Shoaib has not opened his bowels since 20.11.12	Shoaib will have opened his bowels within 24 hours of admission to the ward (i.e. 23.11.12) Shoaib will be having daily bowel movements by time of discharge	(a) Nursing team to increase mobility as per agreed action plan above (problem 2) (b) Nursing team to encourage Shoaib to enhance intake of dietary fibre (e.g. vegetables with main meals). Nutritional intake to be ascertained and recorded by registered nurse since 20.11.12 on each shift (c) Nurses to evaluate the effectiveness of the above interventions using goals and baselines by 23.11.12 (*Final evaluation*)
4.	Shoaib states that he is having difficulty sleeping due to anxiety **Baseline:** about 2 hours sleep per night. 'Worry' scale 8 at worst, 6 at best	Shoaib will sleep for 8 hours per night by 24.11.12 'Worry' scale to be 4 or less by 24.11.12	(a) Nursing staff to offer earplugs to reduce environmental noise (b) Night nursing team to encourage Shoaib to take night sedation on 22.11.12 and 23.11.12 (c) Registered nursing staff to monitor sleep pattern in association with Shoaib and record (*Recheck and ongoing evaluation*) (d) Nurse to evaluate effectiveness of the above interventions using goals and baselines on 24.11.12 (*Final evaluation*)

5. Shoaib states that he is anxious about the fact that he has suffered an MI, and has expressed fears about his future lifestyle, including financial and sexual concerns

Baselines

On a scale (0–10), Shoaib indicates that his 'worry' level is 8

Shoaib believes he will not be able to return to work, and will suffer financially as a result. He also believes that sexual relations with his wife may not be possible

'Worry' scale to be 2 or less by 26.11.12

(a) Nursing staff to give explanations about condition and treatment at every opportunity and encourage Shoaib to ask questions

(b) Nursing team to keep Shoaib's family informed and involved in care wherever possible

(c) Registered nurse to refer Shoaib to cardiac rehabilitation team on 23.11.12

(d) Nursing staff to give Shoaib time to discuss concerns in private, involving Shoaib's family if he so wishes

(e) Nursing staff to offer health education literature for Shoaib to read in his own time

(f) Nursing staff to work with cardiac rehabilitation team to reinforce potential for return to normal functioning

(g) 'Worry' score to be monitored daily by registered nurse and recorded (*Recheck and ongoing evaluation*)

(h) Nurse to evaluate effectiveness of the above interventions on 26.11.12 (*Final evaluation*)

---

6. Without lifestyle modification, and an appropriate medication regime, Shoaib is at high risk of future cardiac events

Baselines

(a) Shoaib smokes 30 cigarettes per day (recommendation is to give up entirely)

(b) Shoaib's BMI is 32 (recommended maximum is 25)

(c) Shoaib's total cholesterol is 6.4mmol/l (recommended is <4.0), LDL 4.3mmol/l (recommended <2.0mmol/l), HDL 1 mmol/l (recommended >1.15 mmol/l)

(d) Shoaib has been commenced on aspirin, Clopidogrel, a beta-blocker, an ACE inhibitor and a statin

(a) Shoaib will give up smoking immediately

(b) Shoaib will plan to lose two stone in weight within 12 months (BMI to 28)

(c) By six months post-discharge Shoaib's total cholesterol will decrease to 4.0 mmol/l, and LDL cholesterol to 2.0 mmol/l

(d) Shoaib will be able to explain the need for, and adhere to, his medication regime by 24.11.12

(a) Nursing team to refer Shoaib to community smoking cessation team on 23.11.12

(b) Nursing team to refer Shoaib to a dietician for dietary advice on 23.11.12

(c) Nursing team to discuss goals a–c with Shoaib and family prior to discharge to ensure ownership of targets

(d) Nursing and medical team to discuss reasons for secondary prevention medication regime with Shoaib prior to discharge

(e) Cardiac rehabilitation team to liaise with primary care practitioners prior to Shoaib's discharge to discuss targets

(f) Nurse to evaluate effectiveness of the above interventions using goals and baselines in relation to goal (d) on 24.11.12 (*Final evaluation*)

Evaluation of progress

Date	Care delivered (use intervention number from care plan)	Evaluation of care
23.11.2012 1500	1(abcfg), 2(abcd), 3(abc), 4(d), 5(abcdeg), 6(ab)	+ Shoaib has not reported breathlessness, dizziness or pain of any sort + Vital signs have remained within normal parameters throughout the day – values at 14:00 were blood pressure 120/70mmHg, pulse 70 bpm, respiratory rate 12 breaths per minute + No additional bruising or swelling in right groin + Shoaib has been reminded of the importance of reporting any pain, dizziness or breathlessness + Nil abnormal detected in dipstick of urine + Shoaib is now mobilising around the bed areas and to and from the toilet in line with the post-MI mobility plan + Shoaib is remembering to carry out gentle leg exercises when in bed + Referral to the cardiac rehabilitation team was made at 11:00 on 23 November + Shoaib has eaten a full breakfast and lunch today. He is drinking tea and water regularly + Bowels were opened at 09:00 with no difficulty. Soft brown stool, with no occult blood detected + Shoaib reports that he slept well last night following medication (see this morning's evaluation) + Shoaib states that he feels 'much less tired' than yesterday + Shoaib's family are visiting at present, and have been given a full update on progress + Shoaib has requested, and been given, a range of reading material about heart disease, which he and his family are going to discuss + Shoaib's anxiety level at 14:00 was 4 (on a scale of 0–10) + Referrals have been made to community smoking cessation team and hospital dietician this morning

References and bibliography

Aggleton P, Chalmers H (2000) *Nursing Models and Nursing Practice*, 2nd ed. Basingstoke: Macmillan Press.

Allen D (1998) Record-keeping and routine nursing practice: the view from the wards. *Journal of Advanced Nursing* 27: 1223–1230.

Anthony D, Parboteeah S, Saleh M, Papanikolaou P (2008) Norton, Waterlow and Braden scores: a review of the literature and a comparison between the scores and clinical judgement. *Journal of Clinical Nursing* 17 (5): 646–653.

Anthony D, Parboteeah S, Saleh M, Papanikolaou P (2010) Do risk assessment scales for pressure ulcers work? *Journal of Tissue Viability* 19(4): 132–136.

August-Brady M (2000) Prevention as intervention. *Journal of Advanced Nursing* 31(6): 1304–1308.

Baldwin B, Longhurst B, Smith G *et al*. (2003) *Introducing Cultural Studies*. Harlow: Pearson Prentice Hall.

Bandolier (2003) On care pathways. *Bandolier Forum*, July, 1–12.

Barrett D (2006) Disease prevention and rehabilitation. In Barrett D, Gretton M, Quinn T (eds) *Cardiac Care: An Introduction for Healthcare Professionals*. Chichester: John Wiley & Sons, pp. 19–31.

Beauchamp T, Childress J (2001) *Principles of Biomedical Ethics*, 5th ed. Oxford: Oxford University Press.

Beck C (1999) Content validity exercises for nursing students. *Journal of Nursing Education* 38(3): 133–135.

Bee H, Boyd D (2006) *The Developing Child*, 11th ed. New York: Harper Collins.

Benner P (1984) *From Novice to Expert*. Menlo Park: Addison Wesley.

Bjelland I, Dahl A, Haug T *et al*. (2002) The validity of the Hospital Anxiety and Depression Scale. An updated literature review. *Journal of Psychosomatic Research* 52: 69–77.

Björvell C, Wredling R, Thorell-Ekstrand I (2003) Prerequisites and consequences of nursing documentation in patient records as perceived by a group of registered nurses. *Journal of Clinical Nursing* 12: 206–214.

Buka P (2008) *Patients' Right, Law and Ethics for Nurses. A Practical Guide*. London: Hodder Arnold.

Campbell H, Hotchkiss R, Bradshaw N, Porteous M (1998) Integrated care pathways. *British Medical Journal* 316: 133–137.

Carpenito L (2000) *Nursing Diagnosis: Application to Clinical Practice*, 8th ed. Philadelphia: Lippincott.

Carpenito-Moyet L (2005) *Understanding the Nursing Process: Concept Mapping and Care Planning for Students*. Philadelphia: Lippincott, Williams & Wilkins.

Cavanagh S (1991) *Orem's Model in Action*. Basingstoke: Macmillan.

Cheevakasemsook A, Chapman Y, Karen F, Davies C (2006) The study of nursing documentation complexities. *International Journal of Nursing Practice* 12: 366–374.

Christenson P, Kenney J (1995) *Nursing Process; Application of Conceptual Models,* 4th ed. St Louis: CV Mosby.

Cox T (1978) *Stress*. Basingstoke: Macmillan.

Cutcliffe J, Barker P (2004) The Nurses' Global Assessment of Suicide Risk (NGASR): developing a tool for clinical practice. *Journal of Psychiatric and Mental Health Nursing* 11: 393–400.

De Luc K (2000) Care pathways: an evaluation of their effectiveness. *Journal of Advanced Nursing* 32(2): 485–496.

Department of Health (2004) Choosing Health: Making Healthy Choices Easier. London: The Stationery Office.

Department of Health (2006) Our Health, Our Care, Our Say: A New Direction for Community Services. London: The Stationery Office.

Department of Health (2010) Excellence and Equity: Liberating the NHS. London: The Stationery Office

Dimond B (2011) *Legal Aspects of Nursing,* 6th ed. Harlow: Pearson Education.

Dy S, Garg P, Nyberg D *et al.* (2005) Critical pathway effectiveness: assessing the impact of patient, hospital care, and pathway characteristics using qualitative comparative analysis. *Health Services Research* 40(2): 499–516.

Eby M (2000) The challenges of being accountable. In Brechin A, Brown H, Eby M (eds) *Critical Practice in Health and Social Care.* London: Sage Publications, pp. 187–208.

Ellershaw J, Murphy D (2005) The Liverpool Care Pathway (LCP) influencing the UK national agenda on care of the dying. *International Journal of Palliative Nursing* 11(3): 132–134.

El-Radhi A (2008) Why is the evidence not affecting the practice of fever management? *Archives of Disease in Childhood*. 93: 918–920.

Erikson E (1980) *Identity and the Life Cycle*. New York: Norton.

Fawcett J (1984) *Analysis and Evaluation of Conceptual Models of Nursing*. Philadelphia: Davis.

Ferguson G, Hildman T, Nichols B (1987) The effect of nursing care planning systems on patient outcomes. *Journal of Nursing Administration* 17: 30–36.

Ford P, Walsh M (1995) *New Rituals for Old. Nursing through the Looking Glass*. Oxford: Butterworth Heinemann.

Gibbons B (1998) Selecting healthcare assessment tools: putting issues of validity and reliability into a wider context. *Nurse Researcher* 5(3): 5–15.

Gibson F, Cargill J, Allison J *et al.* (2006) Establishing content validity of the oral assessment guide in children and young people. *European Journal of Cancer* 42(12); 1817–1825.

Gimenez J (2007) *Writing for Nursing and Midwifery Students*. Houndmills: Palgrave Macmillan.

Green S, Watson R (2006) Nutritional screening and assessment tools for older adults: literature review. *Journal of Advanced Nursing* 54: 477–490.

Gunstone S, Robinson J (2006) Developing an integrated care pathway in dementia. *Mental Health Practice* 10(2): 35–37.

Hale C, Crofts L, Stokoe L (1999) Managed care, case management and multidisciplinary pathways of care: a selective review for the RCN R&D priority-setting exercise. *Nursing Times Research* 4(5): 366–376.

Hartigan I, O'Mahony D (2011) The Barthel Index: comparing inter-rater reliability between nurses and doctors in an older adult rehabilitation unit. *Applied Nursing Research* 24(1): e1–7.

Health Service Ombudsman (2000) *Errors in the Care and Treatment of a Young Woman with Diabetes.* Available from: www.ombudsman.org.uk/improving_services/special_reports/ hsc/diabetes/diabetes_summary.html.

Health Service Ombudsman (2005) *Failure to Treat a Myeloma Patient Adequately and Inadequate Nursing Documentation.* Available from: www.ombudsman.org.uk/improving_services/selected_cases/HSC/ic0403/e1635.html.

Hogston R, Marjoram (2006) *Foundations of Nursing Practice: Leading the Way,* 3rd ed. Basingstoke: Palgrave Macmillan.

Holland K, Jenkins J, Solomon J, Whittam S (2008) *Applying the Roper-Logan-Tierney Model in Practice,* 2nd ed. Edinburgh: Churchill Livingstone.

Humphries D, Heans S (2004) Educating the future workforce: building the evidence about interprofessional learning. *Journal of Health Services Research and Policy* 9(1): 24–27.

Ilag L, Kronick S, Ernst R *et al.* (2003) Impact of a critical pathway on inpatient management of diabetic ketoacidosis. *Diabetes Research and Clinical Practice* 62: 23–32.

Irving K, Treacy M, Scott A (2006) Discursive practices in the documentation of patient assessments. *Journal of Advanced Nursing* 53(2): 151–159.

Jefferies D, Johnson M, Griffiths R (2010) A meta-study of the essentials of quality documentation. *International Journal of Nursing Practice.* 16; 112–124.

Jones A (2007) Admitting hospital patients: a qualitative study of an everyday nursing task. *Nursing Inquiry* 14(3): 212–223.

Kelly J (2005) Inter-rater reliability and Waterlow's pressure ulcer risk assessment tool. *Nursing Standard* 19 (32): 86–92.

Laitinen H, Kaunonen M and Åstedt-Kurki P (2010) Patient-focused nursing documentation expressed by nurses. *Journal of Clinical Nursing* 19: 489–497.

Lee C (2006) Nurses' perceptions of their documentation experiences in a computerized nursing care planning system. *Journal of Clinical Nursing* 15: 1376–1382.

Lee T, Chang P (2004) Standardised care plans: experiences of nurses in Taiwan. *Journal of Clinical Nursing* 13: 33–40.

Mahoney F, Barthel D (1965) Functional evaluation: the Barthel Index. *Maryland State Medical Journal* 14: 56–61.

Martin A, Hinds C, Felix M (1999) Documentation practices of nurses in long-term care. *Journal of Clinical Nursing* 8: 345–352.

Mason C (1999) Guide to practice or 'load of rubbish'? The influence of care plans on nursing practice in five clinical areas in Northern Ireland. *Journal of Advanced Nursing* 29(2): 380–387.

McSherry W (2007) *The Meaning of Spirituality and Spiritual Care Within Nursing and Health Care Practice*. London: Quay Books.

Middleton S, Roberts E (2000) *Integrated Care Pathways: A Practical Approach to Implementation*. Edinburgh: Butterworth Heinemann.

Neuman B (2010a) Betty Neuman's Autobiography and Chronology of the Development and Utilization of the Neuman Systems Model. In Neuman B, Fawcett J (eds) *The Neuman Systems Model*, 5th ed. Upper Saddle River: Prentice Hall.

Neuman B (2010b) The Neuman Systems Model. In Neuman B, Fawcett, J (eds) *The Neuman Systems Model* 5th ed. Upper Saddle River: Prentice Hall.

Neuman B, Fawcett J (2002) *The Neuman Systems Model*, 4th ed. Upper Saddle River: Prentice Hall.

Newton C (1991) *The Roper-Logan-Tierney Model in Action*. Basingstoke: Macmillan Press.

NHSE (1999) *For the Records: Managing Records in NHS Trusts and Health Authorities HSC 199/53 1999*. London: NHSE.

Nursing and Midwifery Council (2003) *Professional Conduct Annual Report 2002–2003*. London: Nursing and Midwifery Council.

Nursing and Midwifery Council (2005) *NMC Fitness to Practice Annual Report 2004–2005*. London: Nursing and Midwifery Council.

Nursing and Midwifery Council (2007) *Standards for Medicines Management*. London: Nursing and Midwifery Council.

Nursing and Midwifery Council (2008) *The Code: Standards of Conduct, Performance and Ethics for Nurses and Midwives*. London: Nursing and Midwifery Council.

Nursing and Midwifery Council (2009a) *Record Keeping: Guidance for Nurses and Midwives*. London: Nursing and Midwifery Council.

Nursing and Midwifery Council (2009b) *Fitness to Practice Annual Report 1st April 2008– 31st March 2009*. London: Nursing and Midwifery Council.

Nursing and Midwifery Council (2010a) Guidance *on Professional Conduct for Nursing and Midwifery students*. London: Nursing and Midwifery Council.

Nursing and Midwifery Council (2010b) *Standards for Pre-registration Nursing Education*. Available from: http://standards.nmc-uk.org/PreRegNursing/Pages/Introduction.aspx.

Nursing and Midwifery Council (2010c) *Essential skills clusters (2010) and guidance for their use (guidance G7.1.5b)* Available from: http://standards.nmc-uk.org/Documents/ Annexe3_%20ESCs_16092010.pdf.

O'Connell B, Myers H, Twigg D, Entriken F (2000) Documenting and communicating patient care: are nursing care plans redundant? *International Journal of Nursing Practice* 6: 276–280.

Oliver D, Papaionnou A, Giangregorio L et al (2008) A systematic review and meta-analysis of studies using the STRATIFY tool for prediction of falls in hospital patients: how well does it work? *Age and Ageing* 37(6): 621–627.

Orem DE (2001) *Nursing: Concepts of Practice*, 5th ed. St Louis: CV Mosby.

Parahoo K (2006) *Nursing Research. Principles, Process and Issues*, 2nd ed. Basingstoke: Palgrave MacMillan.

Pearson A, Vaughan B, Fitzgerald M (2005) *Nursing Models for Practice*, 3rd ed. Edinburgh: Butterworth Heinemann.

Pudner R (2005) *Nursing the Surgical Patient*, 2nd ed. London: Elsevier.

Reinert D, Allen J (2007) The Alcohol Use Disorders Identification Test: an update of research findings. *Alcoholism: Clinical and Experimental Research* 31(2): 185–199.

Rice L, Raizer J, Grimm S (2010) Vitamin D (Vit-D) deficiency is prevalent among patients with glioma brain tumors. *Oncology Nursing Forum* 37(6): E427.

Richmond J, Wright M (2006) Development of a constipation risk assessment scale. *Journal of Orthopaedic Nursing* 10, 186–197.

Riley K (1998) Paving the way. *Health Service Journal*, 26 March: 30–31.

Roper N, Logan W, Tierney A (1996) *The Elements of Nursing,* 4th ed. Edinburgh: Churchill Livingstone.

Roper N, Logan W, Tierney A (2000) *The Roper Logan Tierney Model of Nursing.* Edinburgh: Churchill Livingstone.

Rotter T, Kinsman L, James EL, *et al.* (2010) Clinical pathways: effects on professional practice, patient outcomes, length of stay and hospital costs. *Cochrane Database of Systematic Reviews*: 2010 (3).

Sahib El-Randhi A (2008) Management of fever in paediatric practice. *Nurse2Nurse* 4.

Savage J, Moore L (2004) *Interpreting Accountability.* Oxford: RCN Institute.

Schon DA (1987) *Educating the Reflective Practitioner: Towards a New Design for Teaching and Learning in the Professions.* San Francisco: Jossey-Bass.

Schoonhoven L, Haalboom J, Bousema M *et al.* (2002) Prospective cohort study of routine use of risk assessment scales for prediction of pressure ulcers. *British Medical Journal* 325: 797–801.

Skalski C, DiGerolamo L, Gigliotti E (2006) Stressors in five client populations: Neuman systems model-based literature review. *Journal of Advanced Nursing* 56(1): 69–78.

Smith J, Forster A, Young J (2006) Use of the 'STRATIFY' falls risk assessment in patients recovering from acute stroke. *Age and Ageing* 35: 138–143.

Tierney A (1998) Nursing models: extant or extinct? *Journal of Advanced Nursing* 28(1): 77–85.

Urquhart C, Currell R, Grant MJ, Hardiker NR (2009) Nursing record systems: effects on nursing practice and health care outcomes. *Cochrane Database of Systematic Reviews*, 2009, Issue 1.

Vernon S (2001) Use of standardised scales in community nursing assessment. *Journal of Clinical Nursing* 15(9): 50–53.

Walsh M (1994) *New Rituals for Old: Nursing through the Looking Glass.* Oxford: Butterworth Heinemann.

Walsh M (1997) Will critical pathways replace the nursing process? *Nursing Standard* 11(52): 39–42.

Walsh M (1998) *Models and Critical Pathways in Clinical Nursing,* 2nd ed. Edinburgh: Bailliére Tindall.

Waltz C, Strickland O, Lenz E (2010) *Measurement in Nursing and Health research*, 4th ed. New York: Springer Publishing Company.

Weatherley ND, Jackson PR (2011) The new Sheffield risk and benefit tables for the elderly. *Quarterly Journal of Medicine* 104(1): 3–12.

Wilson B (2005) Stress. In Montague S, Watson R, Herbert R (eds) *Physiology for Nursing Practice*, 3rd ed. Edinburgh: Elsevier.

Wimpenny P (2002) The meaning of models of nursing to practising nurses. *Journal of Advanced Nursing* 40(3): 346–354.

Wood D, Wray R, Poulter N *et al.* (2005) JBS 2: Joint British Societies' Guidelines on prevention of cardiovascular disease in clinical practice. *Heart* 91 (Suppl V): v1–v52.

Yura H, Walsh M (1967) *The Nursing Process*. Norwalk: Appleton-Century-Crofts.

Yura H, Walsh M (1988) *The Nursing Process*, 5th ed. Norwalk: Appleton & Lange.

Index

Note: **bold numbers** indicate page on which a term is first explained; *italic numbers* show Activity boxes, Practice Example boxes, Figures and Tables.